Caring for Older People in Nursing

Sue Barker

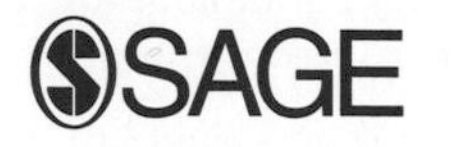
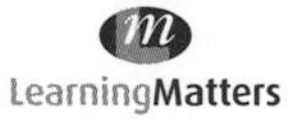

Los Angeles | London | New Delhi
Singapore | Washington DC

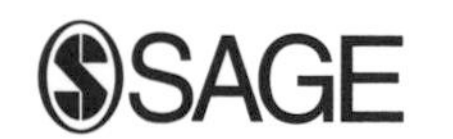

Learning Matters
An imprint of SAGE Publications Ltd
1 Oliver's Yard
55 City Road
London EC1Y 1SP

SAGE Publications Inc.
2455 Teller Road
Thousand Oaks, California 91320

SAGE Publications India Pvt Ltd
B 1/I 1 Mohan Cooperative Industrial Area
Mathura Road
New Delhi 110 044

SAGE Publications Asia-Pacific Pte Ltd
3 Church Street
#10-04 Samsung Hub
Singapore 049483

Editor: Alex Clabburn
Development editor: Caroline Sheldrick
Production controller: Chris Marke
Project management: Swales & Willis Ltd, Exeter, Devon
Marketing manager: Tamara Navaratnam
Cover design: Wendy Scott
Typeset by: C&M Digitals (P) Ltd, Chennai, India
Printed by: Henry Ling Limited at The Dorset Press,
Dorchester, DT1 1HD

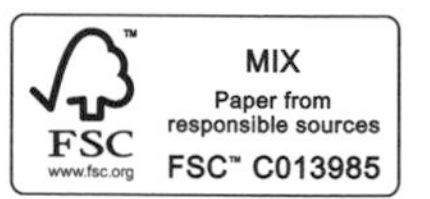

First published 2013

Library of Congress Control Number: 2013947935

British Library Cataloguing in Publication data

A catalogue record for this book is available from the British Library

ISBN 978-1-4462-6762-2
ISBN 978-1-4462-6763-9 (pbk)

Contents

Foreword

As a society we do not value our elders and we tend to make stereotypical judgements about the chronological effects of ageing. Many of these myths and legends are now being dismantled as we hear accounts of octogenarians leading full and active lives – the presenter David Attenborough is an excellent example. In the UK, 12,320 people are now over 100 years old and 650 are over 105 which is a five-fold increase over the last 30 years (ONS). This should be a cause for celebration and a testament to medical science and societal changes. Yet the impact of this growth in the elderly population means major adjustment is needed in our health and welfare provision, social and personal attitudes. What is our role as nurses?

There is a growing recognition that caring for the older person is an integral and major, rather than peripheral, aspect of nursing. Caring for the older person has always been part of nursing and yet it has often been regarded as the Cinderella service. This text provides a timely and refreshing look at giving appropriate, effective and meaningful care to older people.

The editor, Sue Barker, has collected together a series of chapters by respected authors that highlight many facets to deepen your knowledge. The text is underpinned by the concepts of person-centred care and a theory of humanising care to help you develop an even more profound knowledge.

Beginning with an overview of the context of caring for the older person, the text deals with sensitive subjects such as vulnerability, social isolation and loneliness. Specific chapters deepen your knowledge on physical, psychosocial and mental health needs. The concept of wellbeing runs throughout the text and is explored in detail in a dedicated chapter.

We live in a multicultural society in twenty-first century Britain and nurses are expected to keep an open mind and be non-judgemental about cultural mores and ethnicity. This approach is equally important in the care of older persons, and the penultimate chapter provides a clear understanding of the issues in understanding cultural differences and perspectives. Finally, the increasingly important element of interprofessional collaboration is explored with information on the rationale and competencies for interprofessional and interagency care.

You will find this text an engaging, informative and creative read. It is current and will provide you with an excellent resource to understand the needs of older people and improve the quality of their care.

Professor Shirley Bach

Series Editor

About the authors

Dr **Sue Barker** is a registered mental health nurse and chartered psychologist; she works at Bournemouth University in the School of Health and Social Care as a senior lecturer. She is also a member of Bournemouth University Dementia Institute. As part of this she has undertaken consultancy and evaluation work. She has a particular interest in mental and emotional well-being and her PhD explored the emotional care given to women becoming mothers. Sue leads a unit on the mental health nursing programme entitled mental health and well-being in later life.

Michele Board is an adult nurse and has had a broad range of clinical experience, from ward sister to senior nurse, always with a specific focus on nursing the older person. She started lecturing in 2003 on the undergraduate nursing programme, and specialised in themed days on the nursing care of the older person and dementia care.

Michele was appointed as the associate director for the Dementia Institute in February 2013. Since then she has taken the lead in the development of dementia education programmes for health and social care staff working in the NHS and private-sector education.

Michele is also a fellow of the National Institute for Health Research (NIHR) School for Social Care Research, where she is contributing to a research project with the universities of Cambridge, Worcester and York. The aim of the research is to gain a better understanding of how to meet the care and support needs of older people with concurrent sight loss and cognitive impairment and who are living in housing settings (as opposed to care homes).

The research with the NIHR ties in well with Michele's PhD, which she in the process of writing. Her PhD has looked at the meaning of home for baby boomers using an interpretive visual methodology.

Karen Cooper qualified in 1978 and has over 30 years' clinical experience within medicine and care of the older person. Karen was a ward manager for ten years in a rehabilitation setting for older people. She moved into education in 2005, initially as a practice educator, and is currently a lecturer in adult nursing. Her areas of academic and research interests are in practice learning, assessment and mentorship in relation to practitioners' personal and professional practice.

Dr **Lee-Ann Fenge** is Deputy Director of the National Centre for Post-Qualifying Social Work at Bournemouth University. She is a qualified social worker, and has worked in both hospital and local office settings with both adults and children. She has extensive teaching experience at both undergraduate and postgraduate levels. Her research interests concern inclusive research methodologies for engaging with seldom-heard groups, old age and sexuality, and the impact of the recession on older people's well-being.

Rosalind Green is an associate researcher at Bournemouth University and Alexander Technique teacher by background. Her work focuses on the promotion of emdodied knowledge in relation to using the Technique specifically in reduction of background 'noise' when riding. Her work with a variety of adults and children has led to a specific interest in developing a model in which to promote people's understanding of what they are doing with themselves.

Sarah Hean is an associate professor within the well-being and health academic community at Bournemouth University. She is an educational researcher by background, with a keen interest in interprofessional and collaborative practice and learning, specifically that which enhances the quality of life of older people.

Vanessa Heaslip is a senior lecturer in adult nursing; her clinical background was as a district nurse and specialist practitioner for older people. She is aligned to the society and social welfare academic community within Bournemouth University, due to her research interests in hearing the voices of marginalised communities and minority groups. Reflective of these interests, she also sits on the national Mary Seacole award steering group as an independent member, supporting awardees working on projects to enhance the lives of people from ethnic minorities.

Vanessa is also a member of the Bournemouth University Dementia Institute, and works with colleagues providing educational programmes to staff within a variety of clinical settings, challenging them to see beyond a diagnosis of dementia towards seeing the person, as well as developing their understanding of vulnerability. Vanessa has written extensively around the concept of vulnerability, including co-editing a book on vulnerability, and believes that addressing vulnerability is a core aspect of high-quality nursing care.

Dr **Ann Hemingway** is public health research lead with the Academic Centre for Health and Wellbeing at Bournemouth University. Her interests focus on the promotion of sustainable well-being through resident involvement in planning and providing services; and capacity building, particularly in deprived areas. A principal aim of this work is actively to involve residents in well-being improvement and evaluation work. Her career over the last ten years has consisted primarily of managing national and international research and development projects. Ann is guest lecturer in public health/public health nursing at Uppsala University in Sweden and Chair of the European Academy of Caring Science. She is also a member of the leadership group for the UK chapter of Sigma Theta Tau, the international Scholarship Honour Society for Nurses.

Eleanor Jack is an associate lecturer in mental health nursing at Bournemouth University and a member of the well-being and health academic community there. She is an adult and mental health nurse by professional background at junior and senior levels within primary, secondary and tertiary care settings and has also worked as a researcher on a wide variety of research projects for the university since 2001. Eleanor has a keen interest in promoting salutogenic approaches to health and empowerment within the nurse education curricula.

Dr **Janet Scammell** is an associate professor and registered nurse and works for the School of Health and Social Care at Bournemouth University. Her role is professional lead for adult and children's and young people's nursing. Janet is a member of the Mary Seacole award steering group and has mentored several successful awardees over the years. After a career in nursing practice, Janet moved to higher education and has over 20 years' experience as a lecturer and educational leader with undergraduate and postgraduate students in nursing. Janet also facilitates interprofessional education for health and social care students and has led research projects in this area. Janet's current research interests include ethnicity and healthcare practice, including workforce considerations, nursing older people, practice learning and humanisation of care.

Now retired from full-time employment, **Sue Smith** is the principal carer for her 87-year-old mother and has an adult son who has a severe learning disability. She has been involved in multiagency communication within both learning disability (for 37 years) and elderly care (for some 10 years). She worked for over 20 years as public relations/fundraising manager and parent liaison coordinator at the school where her son attended, with some additional involvement in new admissions and marketing. She has been part of the Bournemouth University Carers and Service Users Programme almost since its inception and has enjoyed enormously the variety of opportunities involving prospective social work students. Most recently, she has been involved in end-of-life care for her mother-in-law (diagnosed with advanced, aggressive lung cancer) within a nursing home situation which, although extremely emotional, was nevertheless an experience she felt privileged to be involved in.

Acknowledgements

Sue Barker thanks all at Learning Matters for encouragement, support and patience, particularly Caroline Sheldrick, who has responded to queries quickly and shown sensitivity and support for the authors.

Ann Hemingway would like to thank all the retired nurses who contributed to the discussion about well-being in caring settings included in Chapter 4, for their time, enthusiasm and thoughts.

Eleanor Jack would like to express heartfelt thanks and gratitude to the members, volunteers and staff of the Brendoncare Friendship Clubs who not only gave their time but shared their personal experiences and narratives so freely. During the reflexive and reflective processes inherent within this study, Eleanor was often moved by the sincerity and humility of what she felt privileged to read, hear and see. Much of that experience has informed the writing of her chapter. Grateful thanks go to her mentor Dr Ann Hemingway.

Janet Scammell would like to acknowledge the contribution of four undergraduate nursing students for their case studies in Chapter 8 concerning ageing and care in countries outside the UK. They are: Irina Pavalache; Ida Ngwa Azinnwi; Jitka Mulackova; and Pooja Gurung.

Introduction

About this book

This book is for undergraduate nurses, primarily those working in the adult nursing field, but it will also be helpful for nursing students in the fields of mental health and learning disability. It offers a concise, structured and interactive overview of pertinent areas of practice with older people.

Book structure

This book will explore the opportunities and skills required to look after older people, in the various settings in which nurses will meet them. In Chapter 1 Michele Board and Ann Hemingway set the scene and get you to consider your views of older people, what ageing means and your health expectations. In Chapter 2 Karen Cooper discusses the opportunities in your practice placements where you can develop the skills required to work with and care for older people. Vanessa Heaslip, an adult nurse, has written extensively about vulnerability and considers what this means and the implications for your practice in Chapter 3. Ann Hemingway and Rosalind Green develop the humanisation theory, and discuss the nurse's role in the promotion of well-being in Chapter 4. A significant area of well-being is that of mental well-being, and Sue Barker, a mental health nurse, introduces this in Chapter 7. Lee-Ann Fenge, a social worker by professional background, explores the psychological and sociological aspects of ageing, and Janet Scammell, an adult nurse, sets this in the context of a multicultural society in Chapter 8. Whilst the majority of older people live independently with minimal assistance at home, Eleanor Jack, a mental health nurse, discusses her work around isolation and the impact this has on well-being in Chapter 9.

From our nursing experience we know that caring for older people requires a great deal of skill. Nurses need to be able to assess and work with a group of people who may have more than one need, or comorbidities. Nurses will need to be able to coordinate a multidisciplinary team to be able to assess and meet the complex needs of an individual. In Chapter 5, Michele Board and Karen Cooper, both of whom are adult nurses with extensive nursing experience, discuss how to care for people with the more familiar needs of an older person. Sarah Hean and Sue Smith in Chapter 10 will then highlight the skills required when working interprofessionally.

The book is based on a holistic approach rather than a medical model to the care of older people. We have underpinned each chapter with our own values and beliefs about nursing care, which have been influenced by the humanisation theory. Each chapter can be read independently but we recommend you read it as a developing story.

Requirements for the NMC Standards for Pre-registration Nursing Education and the Essential Skills Clusters

The Nursing and Midwifery Council (NMC) has established standards of competence to be met by applicants to different parts of the register, and these are the standards it considers necessary for safe and effective practice. In addition to the competencies, the NMC has set out specific skills that nursing students must be able to perform at various points of an education programme. These are known as Essential Skills Clusters (ESCs). This book is structured so that it will help you to understand and meet the competencies and ESCs required for entry to the NMC register. The relevant competencies and ESCs are presented at the start of each chapter so that you can clearly see which ones the chapter addresses. There are generic standards that all nursing students, irrespective of their field, must achieve, and field-specific standards relating to each field of nursing, i.e. mental health, children's, learning disability and adult nursing.

This book includes the latest standards for 2010 onwards, taken from Standards for Pre-registration Nursing Education (Nursing and Midwifery Council, 2010).

Learning features

There are a number of activities, case studies, scenarios and further reading or viewing (YouTube) suggestions in each chapter. All of these are linked to the topic covered in the chapter, so in Chapter 1 there is a focus on your own perceptions and views of older people and how they may be different to the realities of nursing. In Chapter 2 the activities relate to your interactions with mentors and how you would undertake clinical tasks whereas others, such as Chapter 6, are more about developing your understanding of the supporting evidence and theories to guide your practice.

Activities

Throughout the book you will find activities in the text that will help you to make sense of, and learn about, the material being presented by the authors. Some activities ask you to reflect on aspects of practice, or your experience of it, or the people or situations you encounter. Reflection is an essential skill in nursing, and it helps you to understand the world around you and often to identify how things might be improved. Other activities will help you develop key skills, such as your ability to think critically about a topic in order to challenge received wisdom, or your ability to research a topic and find appropriate information and evidence, and to make decisions using that evidence in situations that are often difficult and time-pressured. Finally, communication and working as part of a team are core to all nursing practice, and some activities will ask you to carry out group activities or think about your communication skills to help develop these.

All the activities require you to take a break from reading the text, think through the issues presented and carry out some independent study, possibly using the internet. Where appropriate, there are sample answers presented at the end of each chapter, and these will help you to understand more fully your own reflections and independent study. Remember, academic study will always require independent work; attending lectures will never be enough to be successful on your programme, and these activities will help to deepen your knowledge and understanding of the issues under scrutiny and give you practice in working on your own.

You might want to think about completing these activities as part of your personal development plan (PDP) or portfolio. After completing the activity, write it up in your PDP or portfolio in a section devoted to that particular skill, then look back over time to see how far you are developing. You can also do more of the activities for a key skill that you have identified a weakness in, which will help build your skill and confidence in this area.

Chapter 1
The context of nursing older people

Michele Board and Ann Hemingway

NMC Standards for Pre-registration Nursing Education

This chapter will address issues within all four domains of the pre-registration nursing competencies but most significantly the following competencies:

Domain 1: Professional values

2. All nurses must practise in a holistic, non-judgmental, caring and sensitive manner that avoids assumptions, supports social inclusion; recognises and respects individual choice; and acknowledges diversity. Where necessary, they must challenge inequality, discrimination and exclusion from access to care.
3. All nurses must support and promote the health, wellbeing, rights and dignity of people, groups, communities and populations. These include people whose lives are affected by ill health, disability, ageing, death and dying. Nurses must understand how these activities influence public health.

Domain 2: Communication and interpersonal skills.

1. All nurses must build partnerships and therapeutic relationships through safe, effective and non-discriminatory communication. They must take account of individual differences, capabilities and needs.
2. All nurses must use a range of communication skills and technologies to support person-centred care and enhance quality and safety. They must ensure people receive all the information they need in a language and manner that allows them to make informed choices and share decision making. They must recognise when language interpretation or other communication support is needed and know how to obtain it.

Domain 4: Leadership, management and team working

1. All nurses must act as change agents and provide leadership through quality improvement and service development to enhance people's wellbeing and experiences of healthcare.
4. All nurses must be self-aware and recognise how their own values, principles and assumptions may affect their practice. They must maintain their own personal and professional development, learning from experience, through supervision, feedback, reflection and evaluation.

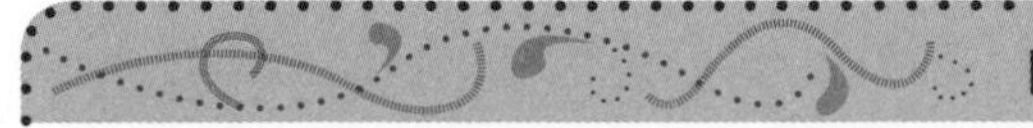

NMC Essential Skills Clusters (ESCs)

This chapter will support the following ESCs:

Cluster: Care, compassion and communication

1. As partners in the care process, people can trust a newly registered graduate nurse to provide collaborative care based on the highest standards, knowledge and competence.

By entry to the register

10. Acts as a role model in promoting a professional image.
11. Acts as a role model in developing trusting relationships, within professional boundaries.
12. Recognises and acts to overcome barriers in developing effective relationships with service users and carers.

2. People can trust the newly registered graduate nurse to engage in person centred care empowering people to make choices about how their needs are met when they are unable to meet them for themselves.

By entry to the register

2:8. Is sensitive and empowers people to meet their own needs and make choices and considers with the person and their carer(s) their capability to care.

3. People can trust the newly registered graduate nurse to respect them as individuals and strive to help them them preserve their dignity at all times.

By entry to the register

3:5. Is proactive in promoting and maintaining dignity.

5. People can trust the newly registered graduate nurse to engage with them in a warm, sensitive and compassionate way.

By entry to the register

6. Anticipates how people might feel in a given situation and responds with kindness and empathy to provide physical and emotional comfort.

Chapter aims

On completion of this chapter you should be able to:

- explain what we mean by 'older people';
- suggest reasons why some people 'age better' than others;
- outline the humanisation theory on the care of individuals, regardless of age.

Introduction

When you told your family and friends you wanted to go into nursing they may well have said, 'You'll make a wonderful nurse'. But some might have added they could not contemplate looking after 'all those old people'! No doubt you will indeed make a wonderful nurse, and in this book we aim to explore how best to care for 'older people'.

During their career all nurses, regardless of their field of nursing, will be involved in the care of older people who will inevitably be part of most families. Therefore it is essential that all nurses have an insight into the unique needs of those aged 65 years and over. The focus of this book is on person-centred care, and introduces you to the humanising theory of care, whereby patients are treated as individuals regardless of their age, ethnic background or diagnosis. Some of you will have chosen a nursing career because you want to care for older people.

The first part of this chapter considers who we are talking about when we say 'older people'. We will look at reasons why some people appear to age 'better' than others and the role nurses can play in supporting healthy ageing. We then introduce humanisation, a nursing theory that underpins the rest of the book. The humanisation theory challenges us to consider each individual, and his or her experiences, and the importance of treating people as individuals regardless of age or illness.

Activity 1.1 *Critical thinking*

Consider what you understand by the term 'older people'. Write down briefly who you think 'older people' are.

As this is a personal reflection, no outline answer is supplied.

In the activity, you may have listed 'My grandparents', 'People aged over 65 years', 'Pensioners', 'People aged over 70 years' or 'Someone older than me!' Regardless of age many people will believe that older people are 'others'. Patients will often say, 'Why have you put me in a bay with old people?', although they are the oldest person, chronologically, in the room. You will also observe some patients who appear to decline rapidly as they withdraw into themselves, and perhaps you think 'so this is old!' Although the day before admission they were living independent lives, they enter an environment where their age becomes significant, and begin to 'feel their age'. These feelings arise because as a society we do not value ageing, and make judgements about people because of their chronological age. But who are older people? It may surprise you to know that the World Health Organization (2013b) defines older people as those aged 60 years or over. The National Service Framework for Older People (Department of Health, 2001b) defines older people as 50 years or over. In this book we will be defining old age as those aged 65 years and over, whilst emphasising that this group is not homogeneous. Just as all those aged between 20 and 60 are not the same, people aged over 60 to 100+ are not all the same either.

Ageing population: time bomb or success story?

The needs of older people are worthy of consideration given the worldwide ageing population. In the European Union in 2060 those aged 65 and over will become a much larger proportion (rising from 17 per cent to 30 per cent of the population), as will the over-80s (rising from 5 per cent to 12 per cent) (European Economy, 2012).

Figures 1.1 and 1.2 are two maps produced by United Nations (2012), which highlight this very well.

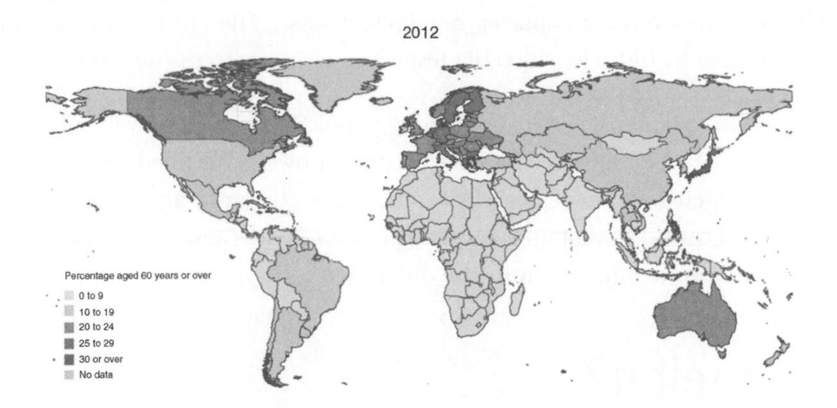

Figure 1.1: Percentage of the total population aged 60 years or over: 2012

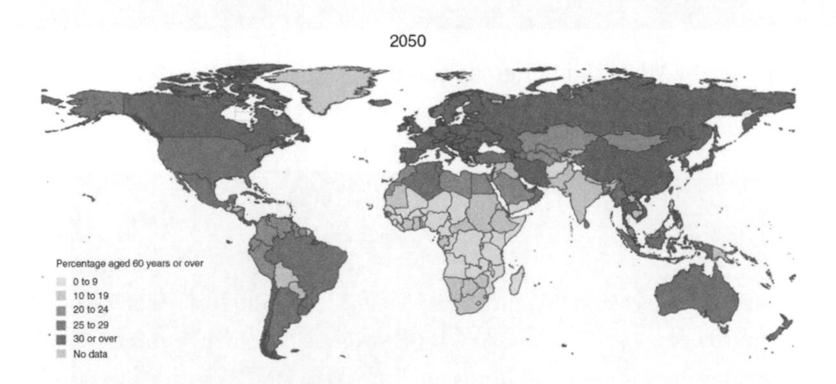

Figure 1.2: Percentage of the total population aged 60 years or over: 2050

Activity 1.2 — ***Critical thinking***

Study these two maps and consider the following:

- Why might there be a younger population in Africa, compared to the UK?
- Why is there a younger population in the USA compared to the UK?
- What are the implications of increased life expectancy for individual people?
- What are the implications of an ageing population for healthcare professionals?
- An outline answer is provided at the end of the chapter.

There are implications of an ageing population both for individuals and health and social care providers. In considering these implications it is important to know what happens as we age. What is normal ageing, and what is common in older age? As healthcare professionals we can have a distorted view of ageing since many of the older and frail people we meet are patients, so by definition with problems. We could think that frailty is in fact synonymous with old age, and not appreciate that the majority of older people live well and independently in their own homes.

Look at the YouTube clip of older athletes at the 2009 Sydney World Masters Games, including track and field, swimming, diving and weight lifting (**http://www.youtube.com/watch?v=4NWZbVb_DLU&feature=player_detailpage#t=0s**). The athletes in the film range in age from their late 50s to 100. The video is a testament to how successfully some people age.

As nurses we need to consider our role in enabling people to stay fit and well and live independent lives, and our role when an older person becomes unwell. We need to challenge negative assumptions about ageing and consider why some people appear to age more successfully than others. Firstly we will consider what normal ageing is, what illness and/or diseases are more common as we age and how we might identify the difference.

What is ageing?

Activity 1.3 *Reflection*

Figure 1.3 shows baby Mary and her great grandmother, Nora. Look carefully at the photo and make a note about how you would define 'ageing'.

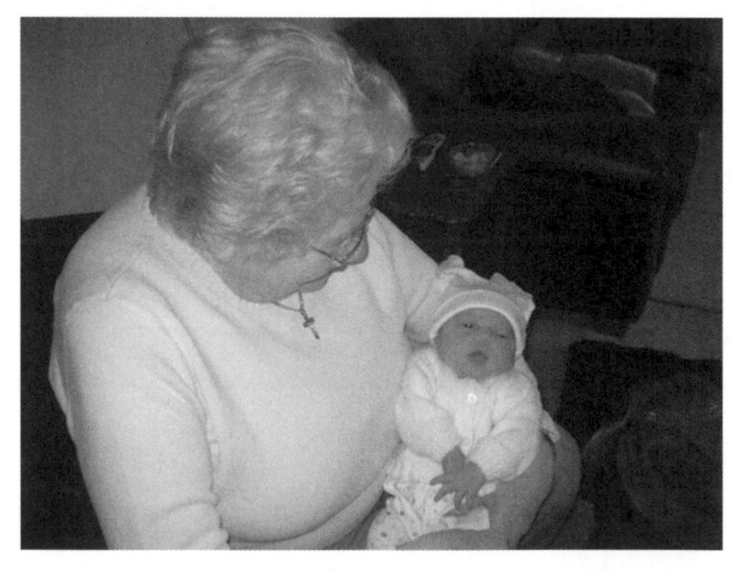

Figure 1.3: Mary and her great-grandmother

As this is a personal reflection, no outline answer is supplied.

The photo is a useful reminder that ageing is happening to us all, part of family life, and therefore relevant for all nurses. Mary was aged just two days old in the photograph, and has already aged considerably since her conception! Robert Butler first coined the term 'ageing' and spoke about how we should celebrate the fact that we now live longer and healthier lives than ever before. He worked throughout his 83 years to change views of older people and was said to have created a new paradigm for old age. Ageing is a real success story which can be attributed to better hygiene, diet and medicine. Ageing is often defined by chronological age, or the passage of time as an individual matures. But chronological age is not everything: it was Mary, not her 80-year-old great-grandmother, who experienced a life-threatening illness hours after this photograph was taken. Fortunately her open-heart surgery was successful and she continues to thrive.

Black's Medical Dictionary (2010) defines ageing as:

> *The result of a combination of natural, largely genetically programmed changes occurring in all body systems. Diseases or injuries may influence these changes, which impair the body's homeostatic mechanisms; environment and lifestyle also affect the ageing process.*

This comprehensive definition refers to the many factors that can influence how successfully we age. Some of these factors have an element of genetic programming, such as cardiovascular disease. However, it also refers to the influence of lifestyle and the environment, which can reduce the genetic effects of, for example, cardiovascular disease but also impact it, such as smoking increasing the risk of cardiovascular disease. The body's ability to maintain homeostasis, or a steady state, is compromised by disease and illness. With normal ageing an individual's reserve capacity to tolerate illness reduces. Like a spare fuel tank in a car, when the spare fuel has been used up, only the main fuel tank is available; with ageing, recovery from illness takes longer and the effects are more damaging because there is no spare fuel.

The definition therefore gives some indications as to why some people may appear to age better than others.

Why do some people appear to age 'better' than others?

In considering this question it may be useful to explore the case study of Nora, Mary's great-grandmother. Read Nora's story and consider what factors are influencing how successful she is ageing.

Case study

Nora is 80 years old. She is the third of four children, and her three siblings live with their spouses in Southern Ireland, where she was born. Her mother died of septicaemia following a burst appendix at 27 years old when Nora was 2 years old. Her father died when he was 80 years old following pneumonia.

(continued)

continued ...

Nora is a mother of 8 children, 18 grandchildren and 8 great-grandchildren. She has been a widow for 18 years and lives alone in a bungalow. Two of her daughters live nearby and pop in most days, helping with some chores (like hoovering under the bed) or gardening. Nora lives independently, driving to do her shopping, preparing a wide range of meals, running her household and personal care completely independently.

Each Wednesday Nora leads a small team of volunteers and prepares lunch for the 'old people' at her local church's luncheon club. She frequently supports people as they undergo chemotherapy, escorting them to the hospital for their day-long treatment. She is very comforting for these people. Sadly, many of Nora's close friends have died. She is a committed Christian, a well-known member of her local church, and her spiritual life is very important to her.

Nora retired from being a community healthcare assistant when she was 60 years old, and at that time she participated in long walks, table tennis, French-speaking classes and swimming. When she was 62 she fell badly and broke her hip. Six years later she was crossing the road, waving at a neighbour, missed the kerb and fell again, resulting in the need for a knee replacement. When she was 72 she was pruning the roses in her raised flower beds and fell as she was getting down; she broke her wrist and tore a ligament in her shoulder. She also had to have her other hip replaced because of osteoporosis.

These falls and joint replacements have severely restricted Nora's mobility; she uses a stick and can only walk short distances. She is frequently in pain because of arthritis in her shoulder and ankle. The subsequent lack of exercise has meant Nora is overweight. This has led to hypertension and high cholesterol. She is on medication for both these conditions. She has had a small vascular event leading to the loss of sight in her right eye. A recent annual review by the practice nurse revealed that her blood pressure and cholesterol were within normal limits; she had lost 4 lb in weight since her last review, but she was missing the company of her peer group.

Activity 1.4 — *Critical thinking*

Read the case study again. What are the factors which influence how successfully Nora is ageing? In what settings might a nurse meet Nora?

An outline answer is provided at the end of the chapter.

Do you think Nora is ageing successfully? Nora will obviously be the best judge of that. Chronological age is obviously key to ageing, but as healthcare professionals we should be working towards a reduced period of morbidity (or disease) in later life, and maintenance of well-being. The latter will be explored throughout the book, but firstly we will briefly consider the theories associated with successful ageing. Nora's story offers a great deal of insight into these various theories.

Nora remains an active member of her church community. As a mother of eight, and retired community healthcare assistant, she has spent a great deal of her time in a caring role. This has continued into later life at the luncheon club, and trips to the hospital. This sense of purpose to her week and the important role she has ties in with the sociological theories of ageing. Parsons (cited in Heath and Schofield, 1999) talks about *role theory* and the sense of purpose and structure that having a role has on an individual's well-being. Nora is also an example of the valuable contribution those aged 60 years and above make in society. Rather than being seen as a burden, older people have significant formal and informal roles as carers, grandparents, voluntary workers, and so on, contributing to a successful society.

Havighurst (1961) also emphasises the importance of activity. Activity theory supports the importance of retired people having a role and regular activities. As nurses we may need to consider how we support individuals as they prepare for retirement, to avoid isolation, boredom and a feeling of not contributing after a lifetime of being valuable members of society. Obviously health and finances may influence what an individual can do, but even people living in a nursing home should be given opportunities to 'contribute' to the running of 'their home'. This could include helping to tidy their room, make cakes, offering hand massages to the staff! Activity, having a role and sense of purpose, can lead to successful ageing.

Having a family is also a significant factor in successful ageing. Two of Nora's daughters visit her daily. This additional support will enable Nora to remain in her own home. Having family around to undertake activities of daily living, such as meals, shopping, cleaning and general maintenance, is key to enabling older people to remain in their own home as they age. This is an important consideration if you meet a person with no family and no social network to give support at home. We also need to bear in mind the impact that increasing divorce rates and remarriage or new relationships have on family relationships and who will help look after grandparents.

With an increasing number of older adults, especially those aged 80 years and over, the need for additional support to enable them to remain in the community is relevant for health and social care staff. The role of caring for a relative invariably falls to daughters. Yet the well-being of this group of women may also need to be considered as they come into contact with healthcare professionals. These women may be earning the family's keep, and have other family to support, perhaps grandchildren, and juggling all these roles can be demanding and stressful.

It is never too late to exercise, and the benefits of exercise continue throughout life. The YouTube clip about older athletes (**http://www.youtube.com/watch?v=4NWZbVb_DLU&feature=player_detailpage#t=0s**) is testament to the benefits of exercise at any age. Nora undertakes limited exercise. Robert Butler suggested the key to successful ageing was ensuring the quadriceps muscles in the thighs were regularly worked. If these remained strong, he argued, you can safely lower yourself into a chair and stand up from sitting, so you can go to the toilet, make a cup of tea, and so on. Regular exercise helps reduce cholesterol and blood pressure, reduce weight and increase well-being. As nurses we must respect individuals' right to choose if, after being informed of the importance of exercise, they choose not to engage. However, we should try hard to offer plenty of choices.

The loss of a spouse, through death or divorce, and of friendship groups can contribute to loneliness, isolation and depression in later life. Although depression was not identified by the practice nurse, Nora did admit to feeling lonely and a bit isolated because her peer group, specifically her close friends, had died. Nurses need to be alert to the support an individual may require having experienced numerous losses. Biley et al. (2011, p. 8) discovered that loss in later life can be multiple:

> *Losing the ability to easily share aspects of life with another (often following the loss of a life partner) and/or others; a (negative) alteration in mobility; the experience of bereavement and the need to learn new life skills (that had previously been undertaken by the deceased); changes in health; a recognition, in the words of one participant, that 'life shrinks' (as a result of altered financial status, bereavement, an altered social network and reduced mobility – often in combination); and finally, the acknowledgement of the need 'to ask' (for advice and help).*

The poignancy of 'life shrinks', as mentioned to myself (Board) as part of this piece of research, reinforced the important role we as nurses have to ensure we take into account older people's social history when assessing them, to help identify where we can intervene and offer additional support.

Nora's strong faith undoubtedly offers her comfort and a sense of purpose. Those without such a faith may find this comfort and purpose through other means, in a way that is meaningful for them. It can be significant for an individual, and assessment and acknowledgement of this should be made by nursing staff.

Focusing on Nora's health needs would not reveal all the other factors that contribute to well-being and whether she is ageing successfully or not. As nurses we may meet Nora in hospital, in a GP practice, or as a member of a family. A recognition of the complexity of healthy ageing will enable us to support Nora in the most appropriate way for her. A focus on her obvious health needs would mean we would ignore the complexity of her needs. But we do need to consider her physical health needs, and how these might impact upon her ageing successfully.

Biological theories of ageing

A great deal of research is being undertaken to explore the various biological features of ageing. For example, it is widely accepted that a predictor of longevity is the age your parents died, suggestive of a genetic influence. Nora's siblings are all alive. Her father lived until he was 80, and although her mother died at a young age, advances in medicine now would have made that less likely.

These programmed theories of ageing note that the human species has a maximum life span. There are genes that turn on and off during the life span. Evidence to support these theories is the existence of life changes, such as puberty and menopause. There are the non-genetic or wear-and-tear theories of ageing. These attribute ageing to progressive cell damage caused by the internal and external environment. With age, cells change, impacting upon their effectiveness, so poor ageing is a result of progressive damage.

The main causes of cell damage have been very well studied, the major factors being oxygen (or free radical damage) and glucose-mediated damage (causing damage to the protein in cells), paradoxically the molecules needed to sustain life. Cells die and/or become stiffer with increasing age.

Random damage is not everything; there are links between theories of ageing and common diseases involving lifestyle factors.

For example, Nora has hypertension and has had a small vascular event leading to the loss of sight in her eye. Protein damage to the blood vessel walls causes them to lose their elasticity, resulting in hypertension. However, a high-cholesterol diet and reduced exercise cause the build-up of fatty plaques on the arterial walls, narrowing the lumen and increasing blood pressure and becoming a risk factor for stroke and myocardial dysfunction. The damage to the inner lining of the arterial wall, or endothelium, is made worse by oxidative damage, preventing cell repair. So, as a consequence of lifestyle and biological changes, Nora needs medication to reduce any further risk of a cardiovascular event.

Nora also has osteoporosis. Osteoporosis is a condition characterised by low bone mass and increased bone fragility, putting patients at risk of fractures, which are major causes of morbidity in older people. Being postmenopausal, female and having limited exercise are factors which have increased Nora's risk of having osteoporosis. There are non-modifiable (genetic) and modifiable (lifestyle) factors associated with ageing. Genetic factors have been linked to various diseases, including Alzheimer's disease and cardiovascular disease; however, risk for cardiovascular disease can be accelerated by lifestyle factors such as smoking. Your genetic make-up will also offer clues to your life expectancy, and the life span of your parents may give you a clue as to your own life span (Hall, 2013). Lifestyle factors such as diet, exercise, alcohol consumption and smoking are well-known factors that influence healthy ageing. It is never too late to advise an older person to adopt positive lifestyle choices.

In other words, successful ageing, in relation to preventing fractures and cardiovascular disease, can be improved with weight-bearing exercise, good diet (calcium and low fat), reduced alcohol and not smoking. This would be especially relevant if there is a genetic risk factor for these diseases in a family.

Activity 1.5 — ***Critical thinking***

Look at Table 1.1 and consider the role nurses play in supporting individuals to reduce the risk of modifiable aspects of ageing. Note the positive impact of exercise and balanced diet.

(continued)

continued ...

Aspect of ageing		Means of modifying the aspect
Ageing skin	→	Sun avoidance
Cardiac reserve	→	**Exercise**, non-smoking
Dental decay	→	Prophylaxis, **diet**
Elevated blood pressure	→	**Salt limitation, weight control, exercise**
Glucose tolerance	→	Weight control, **exercise, diet**
Intelligence tests	→	**Training,** practice
Memory	→	**Training,** practice
Osteoporosis	→	Weight-bearing **exercise, diet**
Physical endurance	→	**Exercise, weight control**
Physical strength	→	**Exercise**
Pulmonary reserve	→	**Exercise**, non-smoking
Reaction time	→	**Training**, practice
Serum cholesterol	→	**Diet**, weight control, **exercise**
Social ability	→	Practice

Table 1.1: Modifiable aspects of ageing

As this is a personal reflection, no outline answer is supplied.

Nurses need to be very skilled when looking after an older person, whose needs are often complex and whose life story may be rich. Looking after an older person is like putting together a jigsaw puzzle: a team approach helps this assessment and is one of the pleasures of specialising in nursing this age group. Effective communication between the various team members is essential if we are going to meet the unique needs of the unique individuals we care for. The humanisation theory of nursing suggests a framework that enables us to see the unique individual experience of those you will be caring for. A humanising approach to care can ensure the experience of the individual is at the heart of care delivery. It is to this humanising theory of nursing that we now turn.

Humanisation theory of nursing

Throughout this book we advocate the 'value framework for practice', as proposed by Todres et al. (2009), because of its relevance for nursing older people. This proposed framework introduces humanising values to influence practice and research. The framework articulates eight specific constituents of what it is to be human, called 'dimensions'. The dimensions constitute a value base for considering the potentially humanising and dehumanising elements in care systems and interactions. This framework is useful when considering nursing practice, particularly in relation to developing new knowledge of what is both humanising and dehumanising.

In this section of the chapter we look at each dimension of the framework, with a reflection on each dimension in relation to nursing practice. There are questions which have no right or wrong answers: they are intended to help you think about each dimension in relation to your own nursing practice.

Dimensions of what it means to be human

Theory box: The dimensions of humanisation (Todres et al., 2009)

Forms of humanisation	Forms of dehumanisation
Insiderness	Objectification
Agency	Passivity
Uniqueness	Homogenisation
Togetherness	Isolation
Sense making	Loss of meaning
Personal journey	Loss of personal journey
Sense of place	Dislocation
Embodiment	Reductionist body

Table 1.2

We will now consider these dimensions individually to explain their meaning further.

Insiderness/objectification

As nurses we need to ensure we never make those we care for feel like objects.

To be human is to experience life in relation to how you are: your feelings, mood and emotions are all a lens through which you experience the world. An approach to nursing which does not focus on a patient's problems but on the person's potential and assets (skills, knowledge, motivation) helps prevent us treating people like objects, problems, needs or 'diseases' (Hemingway, 2012). As nurses we need to see patients as individuals with the potential to be involved and help solve problems rather than as fragmented risks. This is particularly relevant in nursing older people, about whose needs, beliefs, values and abilities we can make negative assumptions.

Activity 1.6 ***Reflection***

- How can you ensure you never make those you care for feel like objects in your practice area?
- What type of attitude do you need to have to ensure this?
- What specific elements of your behaviour are important to ensure this?

An outline answer is provided at the end of the chapter.

Agency/passivity

We need to ensure that we offer and enable choice and freedom for those we care for.

As humans we make choices and are generally held accountable for our actions. We do not commonly see ourselves as passive but we have the potential to live and act within limits (Hemingway et al., 2012). Seeing ourselves as possessing a sense of choice or freedom appears to be linked to our social, physical and mental health (Stansfeld et al., 2002).

It is a mistake to view older people as passive recipients of nursing care or as problems waiting to be solved or treated. Doing so may result in individuals becoming disempowered. We need to maintain a sense of agency (the feeling that we have control and are able to make choices) in those we care for. We need to look for ways to help patients to take matters into their own hands and self-manage and own the way forward for their care.

Activity 1.7 ***Reflection***

- How can you ensure you offer choice and freedom to those you care for in your practice area?
- What type of attitude do you need to have to ensure this?
- What specific elements of your behaviour are important to ensure this?

An outline answer is provided at the end of the chapter.

Uniqueness/homogenisation

We need to ensure that we get to know the patients and their context; we need to focus on building trusting relationships

Our uniqueness as human beings can never be reduced to a list of general characteristics; we are unique in space and time, in relation to our relationships and our context, and this is how we see ourselves (Todres et al., 2009).

In order to classify patients, we often group them as diabetic, smokers, obese, socially isolated, old, confused, for example; in doing so, we ignore their uniqueness. This 'cookie cutter', one-size-fits-all approach to care dissociates individuals from the context of their life (Hemingway, 2012). When we focus on problems within nursing care we should always consider an individual's context, and avoid generalisations that miss the particular characteristics and strengths of that individual. The complexities of life affect our ability to change our health, or self-care behaviour (Harker and Hemingway, 2003). They are therefore essential for us to consider as nurses.

The 6 Cs strategy

The 6 Cs strategy was launched in 2013 by the Chief Nursing Officer for England (Cummings, 2013) as a way of influencing care delivery to ensure compassionate care. Interestingly, the humanisation model ensures that in practice these six areas are experienced by those we care for.

Our Culture of Compassionate Care
NHS
The
6 Cs
1. Care
2. Compassion
3. Competence
4. Communication
5. Courage
6. Commitment

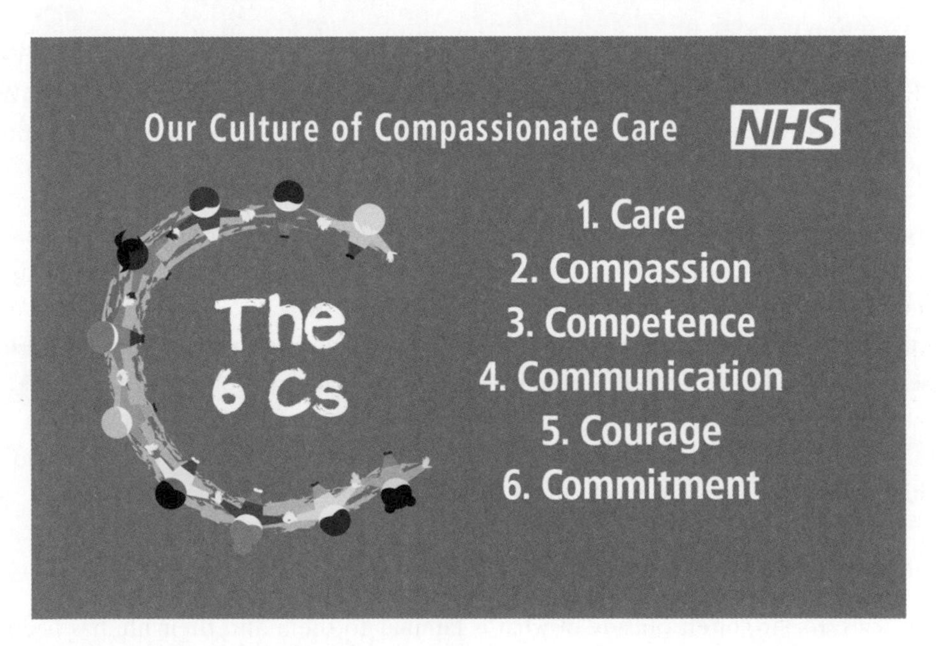

Figure 1.4: The 6 Cs strategy (Cummings, 2013)

As you work through this book, consider how the humanisation model may help enable you to put the 6 Cs into action in practice. The humanisation framework helps to influence our attitudes and behaviour by ensuring that we treat everyone equally as a human being. Having compassion for another person means having empathy and understanding for their situation and a desire to help them; however, we also need to enable this empathy and understanding to inform how we behave in order to influence our attitudes and improve our practice.

Togetherness/isolation

As nurses we need to ensure that we offer those we care for support and the opportunity to build relationships and friendships.

To be human is to be part of a community and to be unique. Social isolation can have a negative impact on our health (Tomaka et al., 2006) whilst negative, destructive relationships may also cause us harm.

Social isolation impacts negatively on outcomes of chronic physical and psychological disease in older people (Drennan et al., 2008). As nurses we need to be acutely aware of the importance of social interaction and the need for patients to be able to trust us. We must check that all our interactions centre on trust and the dignity of all concerned.

Sense making/loss of meaning

We must always explain what is happening and ensure that patients and relatives understand fully their situation and that it makes sense to them in the context of their life.

To be human is to care about the meaning of events and experiences. The immediacy of the search for meaning for many outweighs the significance of the search for statistical truth. We may be unable to make sense of ourselves as part of the top or bottom ten per cent of the population in terms of weight or blood sugar levels or age.

Organisations divide an individual's experiences spatially (ward from outpatients from home care from economic support). Human needs are holistic. When we are counted as a statistic our treatment or prevention opportunities may not make sense because what is 'significant' statistically does not necessarily connect with our human experience. Individuals may indeed help to make sense of their health and well-being by looking at the overall context of their lives, where and how they live, rather than through official articulation of health risks and problems. Nurses need to help individuals to interpret issues in a way that empowers those they care for and builds on existing strengths, enabling involvement in decisions.

Personal journey/loss of personal journey

Those we care for are often outside of what is familiar to them and their life has been interrupted, sometimes dramatically. We need to value their concerns and help them to adapt.

Human beings move through time, and their life course, in a meaningful way; we continually position ourselves in terms of our past, present and future and our context. We are familiar with our past and could be ambivalent, fearful, excited or bored by our future. The experiences that someone has with healthcare are only a part of their life; the interruption or threat caused to this by their illness may cause them great distress, which as nurses we need to be acutely aware of. An excessive emphasis on labelling and treating those we care for negatively as needy or problematic does nothing to enhance their sense of pride and engagement with past, present and future. Indeed, this approach could be conceptualised as disempowering and disabling for individuals (Hemingway, 2012).

Activity 1.8 *Reflection*

- How can you ensure you value the concerns of those you care for and help them to adapt in your practice area?
- What type of attitude do you need to have to ensure this?
- What specific elements of your behaviour are important to ensure this?

An outline answer is provided at the end of the chapter.

Sense of place/dislocation

Healthcare environments can be frightening and confusing places. We need to ensure that through our care of the environment and of our patients we reduce this sense of dislocation.

To be human is to come from a particular place. A sense of home and place is not just a collection of objects or experiences. It offers us security, comfort and familiarity. In addition, spaces need to be understood as potentially providing an environment for bonds and connections between people to flourish (Putnam, 2000). Well-being cannot be separated from the 'place', the atmosphere and 'rhythms' created by the 'built' and natural environment, in all its varied manifestations. The independent effect of place and residence on health and well-being cannot be ignored (Diez Roux, 2001) and arguably the only way to intervene successfully is to be ready to listen to what makes up a sense of home and place for individuals. Indeed, some researchers have articulated the importance of space and architecture as preservers of human dignity, particularly within caring contexts (Martinsen, 2006). Older people often have to move home due to life changes, which may be financial, social or health-related. When we are caring for them we need to ensure that we endeavour at all times to help people feel 'at home' through discovering what matters to them and then through management of the physical, spiritual and social environment.

Embodiment/reductionist view of the body

Every person is equally unique and valuable throughout their life course, and through our behaviour we need to ensure that we treat everyone with respect and dignity.

We experience the world through our bodies in a positive or negative way. An underpinning assumption of the term embodiment is that an individual's biology cannot be understood without considering psychosocial and sociocultural aspects of development (McLaren and Hawe, 2005). An example of this is discrimination in terms of age, race or gender, for instance, which provides evidence for embodiment, whereby the adverse effects get 'under the skin' of individuals and cause poor health (Rayner, 2009). Embodiment relates to how we experience the world, which includes our perceptions of our context and its possibilities, or limits. This may be impacted upon by, for example, our experiences of illness, changes in our body image through ageing or ill health, or our ability to live our life. An excessive emphasis on physiology and tests and not putting the person into his or her wider social context limits our ability to respond to another human being in a caring and dignified way. We need to use language (body and oral) and methods at all times to offer positive perceptions, so we see ourselves and others as creative and able to contribute actively to our own recovery and well-being. Crucially, we need to not make assumptions about older people and recognise the assets of other human beings throughout the course of their lives.

Activity 1.9 *Reflection*

- How can you ensure you treat everyone with respect and dignity and that you don't make assumptions about those you care for in your practice area?
- What type of attitude do you need to have to ensure this?
- What specific elements of your behaviour are important to ensure this?

As this is a personal reflection, no outline answer is supplied.

As nurses, maintaining the best standards of care in our area of practice is our responsibility. Focusing care on what is important to us as human beings enables us always to put this first, to treat everyone as we would wish to be treated and maintain the very best standards of care as a result.

Activities: brief outline answers

Activity 1.2

The study of demography, that is, the study of population, is fascinating. It is particularly relevant for those interested in nursing older people. Why we have an ageing population and the significance for health and social care professionals are worthy of consideration. Health and social care needs, living arrangements and family structures are just some of the factors that will influence healthy ageing. Go to **http://www.ilcuk.org.uk** for more information.

The world maps (Figures 1.1 and 1.2) are interesting because they tell us a lot about the ageing population in the world. Europe has an older population compared to the USA and Africa. The significant feature of this is fertility. European fertility (i.e. the number of babies born) in comparison to the number of older people is lower. So, rather than the population being shaped like a pyramid, that is, more babies (base of the pyramid) and fewer older people, the pyramid shape is changing, with an increasingly fatter top. Look up the population pyramid for your town compared to the rest of the UK on Google. Christchurch, for example, has the oldest population in the UK.

Other factors influencing the shape of the population include migration, and the USA has a higher migration rate of younger people entering and having children, hence they have a younger population than Europe.

In Africa, AIDS and war decrease the proportion of older people in comparison to births, and so at present Africa has a younger population. Access to clean water and medication mean people live longer, but the most influencing factor of an ageing population is fertility.

Activity 1.4

The factors which influence how successfully Nora is ageing include:

- healthy lifestyle, such as balanced diet, adequate exercise;
- positive relationships with others;

- living arrangements;
- finances;
- health, such as absence of pain;
- sense of purpose.

A nurse might meet Nora in the following settings:

- practice nurse;
- out-of-hours service;
- community nurse;
- hospital.

Activity 1.6

This activity asked you to reflect on how you can ensure you don't objectify those you care for. This would mean that you always acknowledge their presence, ask their permission and explain what is happening. In addition you would need to try and put yourself in their shoes and understand how they may be feeling about what is happening to them. For instance, when you explain about their health issue you would do so in a way which acknowledges them as an individual and ask whether they understand and if they have any questions.

The type of attitude that you need to achieve this is empathic, considerate and gentle, which puts patients and their feelings/experience first in your encounters with them. Your behaviour would need to reflect this in how you speak to them, how you touch them and through your body language.

Activity 1.7

You need to ensure you offer choice and freedom wherever possible to those you care for, for instance, in relation to their position, their personal hygiene, their dietary intake and the drinks they have or what they wear, listen to or watch. These may feel like small things for you as a carer but are very important for those being cared for as they may be the only things they feel that they have any say in within a healthcare environment. You need to ask for permission and negotiate what happens with those you care for.

Once again, your attitude needs to be an empathic, considerate, gentle one that puts your patients and their feelings/experience first in your encounters with them. You need to listen to their wishes and comply wherever possible or negotiate a compromise and ensure that you have explained why this is necessary.

Activity 1.8

This activity requires you to think about listening and being patient. You will not be aware of anyone's concerns over anything unless you develop these skills and display them through your behaviour. Take the time to explain things so that those you are caring for understand you. Check their understanding, then take time and allow them to express their concerns; notice their body language, and how they are. Do they appear worried and anxious? Give them the time to share anxieties with you and be patient.

Useful websites

Age UK: http://www.ageuk.org.uk

Information and advice for the elderly about benefits, care, age discrimination and computer courses. Excellent resource for sharing with older people; also links to current research.

Growing Older Research Programme: http://www.growingolder.group.shef.ac.uk

The Growing Older Programme consists of 24 research projects focused on how to extend the quality of life in old age. They were commissioned together as part of a £3.5 million investment by the UK Economic and Social Research Council. They are fascinating projects related to the lives of older people. Research projects include defining and measuring quality of life; inequalities in quality of life; the role of technology and the built environment; healthy and productive ageing; family and support networks; and participation and activity in later life. The research was undertaken between 1999 and 2004.

International Longevity Centre-UK: http://www.ilcuk.org.uk

The International Longevity Centre-UK is the leading think tank on longevity and demographic change. It is an independent, non-partisan think tank dedicated to addressing issues of longevity, ageing and population change. Very interesting reports and papers related to the older person.

Further reading

Heath, H and Schofield, I (1999) *Healthy Ageing: Nursing older people.* London: Mosby.

Interesting and readable book, covering theoretical foundations of ageing; basic biological needs, safety and security, belonging, self-esteem and self-actualisation.

The OU Rethinking Ageing Series has some excellent titles and evidence-based books which are easily readable texts. These are a few:

Bond, J and Corner, L (2004) *Quality of Life and Older People.* Buckingham: Open University Press.

Bytheway, B (1995) *Ageism: Rethinking ageing.* Buckingham: Open University Press.

Kitwood, T (1997) *Dementia Reconsidered: The person comes first.* Buckingham: Open University Press.

Chapter 2
Placement experiences with older people

Karen Cooper

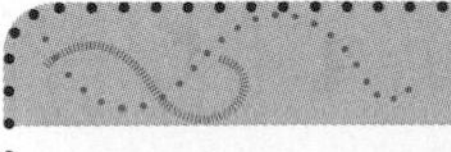

NMC Standards for Pre-registration Nursing Education

Domain 1: Professional values

Generic standard for competence

All nurses must act first and foremost to care for and safeguard the public. They must practise autonomously and be responsible and accountable for safe, compassionate, person-centred, evidence-based nursing that respects and maintains dignity and human rights. They must show professionalism and integrity and work within recognised professional, ethical and legal frameworks. They must work in partnership with other health and social care professionals and agencies, service users, their carers and families in all settings, including the community, ensuring that decisions about care are shared.

Domain 2: Communication and interpersonal skills

Generic standard for competence

All nurses must use excellent communication and interpersonal skills. Their communications must always be safe, effective, compassionate and respectful. They must communicate effectively using a wide range of strategies and interventions including the effective use of communication technologies. Where people have a disability, nurses must be able to work with service users and others to obtain the information needed to make reasonable adjustments that promote optimum health and enable equal access to services.

Domain 3: Nursing practice and decision-making

Generic standard for competence

All nurses must practise autonomously, compassionately, skilfully and safely, and must maintain dignity and promote health and wellbeing. They must assess and meet the full range of essential physical and mental health needs of people of all ages who come into their care. All nurses must also meet more complex and coexisting needs for people in their own nursing field of practice, in any setting including hospital, community and at home. All practice should be informed by the best available evidence and comply with local and national guidelines. Decision-making must be shared with service users, carers and families and informed by critical analysis of a full range of possible interventions, including the use of up-to-date technology.

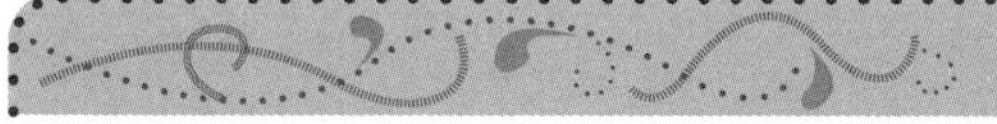

NMC Essential Skills Clusters (ESCs)

This chapter will support all the ESCs, particularly:

Care, compassion and communication

1.12. Recognises and acts to overcome barriers in developing effective relationships with service users and carers.

2.1. Takes a person centred, personalised approach to care.

Organisational aspects of care

9.12. In partnership with the person, their carers and their families, makes a holistic, person centred and systematic assessment of physical, emotional, psychological, social, cultural and spiritual needs, including risk, and together, develops a comprehensive personalised plan of nursing care.

Nutrition and fluid management

27.6. Uses knowledge of dietary, physical, social and psychological factors to inform practice being aware of those that can contribute to poor diet, cause or be caused by ill health.

Chapter aims

By the end of this chapter you will be able to:

- understand the importance of the learning environment in developing knowledge, skills and attitudes required for effective care delivery;
- identify opportunities that will enhance the delivery of person-centred care for older people;
- explore links between theory and practice during placement experiences;
- discuss the role of self and others in achievement of standards of competence.

Below is an extract from a student (Royal College of Nursing, 2008) document discussing working with older people:

> *As a student nurse I love caring for older adults. I find the experience of working with them fulfilling and enriching. They are the teachers and I am the student. From entering their world, sharing laughs and hearing the odd family secret, to blushing when a sweet lady tells me she still enjoys sex with her husband: all of these are held in the sacredness of lived experiences – dreams, disappointments, fuller understandings of truth, body changes and frailty, spirit changes through clarity and wisdom, grace given and grace received and the expectations of life that does not end. And when the time does arrive for them to leave this world, then I hold their hands as they begin their final journey – an honour I*

treasure and hold dear. They have given a lifetime of love to those closest to them and now, in their most vulnerable times, it is their turn to receive compassion. Nursing the older adult is about sharing of a life so richly lived. And the understanding of the complex needs of an individual human being – from helping someone to have a drink of water, to assisting them to walk to the bathroom, to sitting down and listening to their fears.

It is about working with the multidisciplinary team to ensure the patient's independence can be maintained in the outside world. And when it is not possible to return to familiar surroundings then it is about finding places they can call home and receiving the care they so justly deserve. When I have seen a patient smile through mental anguish or physical pain, I feel I have achieved something wonderful.

Introduction

The healthcare needs of the older person are recognised as being the greatest challenge to all practitioners, both nationally and internationally (Nolan et al., 2006b). Today, there are some 600 million people aged 60 and over worldwide; this total will double by 2025 and will reach nearly one and half billion by 2050, with most of the increase in developing countries (World Health Organization, 2011).

The Royal College of Nursing (2008) identifies that older people are the main users of health and social care services, with two-thirds of hospital beds occupied by people over the age of 65 (Bridges et al., 2009). Older people frequently need to be admitted to hospital more often and for longer periods than other age groups, usually with more than one diagnosis or an underlying chronic illness (Barton and May, 2012).

The ageing process leads to physiological, psychological and sociological changes. This can result in older people having more than four diagnoses at the same time, known as multiple pathology (Royal College of Nursing, 2008). With the increase in older people and the multiple pathologies identified, nurses will need to work with increased numbers of older people with mental health problems. The Royal College of Psychiatrists (2005) stated that at any one time up to 60 per cent of older people occupying NHS beds will have mental health needs, mainly dementia, delirium and depression. Nurses therefore need to be skilled in addressing the complex holistic needs of older people. The expectation of the Nursing and Midwifery Council (NMC) (2010) that student nurses develop into knowledgeable, compassionate, critical-thinking, accountable and safe practitioners is clearly necessary given the complex care needs they will encounter.

This chapter will focus on how you can develop your understanding of caring for older people through an exploration of placement experiences. A case study of Molly and Frank, who you will meet again in Chapter 3, and a snapshot of their experience of care will be used as one example of highlighting care needs and how these can be addressed. The scenario related to Molly and Frank is based within a hospital ward but as student nurses you will work with older people in a range of settings, such as nursing homes, community settings and patients' own homes. The knowledge, skills and attitudes that will be discussed throughout the chapter are ones that are transferable to any setting or adult age group and key to your development as a competent practitioner. The first part of this chapter will explore mentoring and the learning environment; the rest of the chapter is structured using the five ESCs, but the first cluster, care, compassion and communication, is considered in most depth as it underpins all other interactions.

Mentoring and the learning environment

Nursing is a practice-based discipline and 50 per cent of current pre-registration nurse education takes place in the clinical setting (Pellatt, 2006). During practice placements student nurses are assigned a mentor for the duration of each clinical experience. A mentor is a nurse who has undergone specific preparation and is defined as one who *facilitates learning, supervises and assesses students in a practice setting* (Nursing and Midwifery Council, 2008a, p. 45). They support student nurses and assess their competence, which is a requirement for entry to the NMC register. Competence is a holistic concept that may be defined as *the combination of skills, knowledge and attitudes, values and technical abilities that underpin safe and effective nursing practice and interventions* (Nursing and Midwifery Council, 2010). Mentors will be assessing the student nurse's practice through observation, discussion and asking questions. They will also encourage reflection on practice, which will help understanding of relevant underpinning knowledge.

Your placements are designed to provide learning opportunities that will advance personal learning and prepare you for registration. A broad range of placement provider organisations, which include NHS and non-NHS settings, such as nursing homes, are used to support you in this aim.

Brown et al. (2008) found that if student nurses experience *enriched environments* then learning experiences can be enhanced. The characteristics of an enriched environment can be understood using the senses framework, which will be discussed later in this chapter. It is a useful means of exploring how care can be used as an analytic lens to understand the older person's needs (Nolan et al., 2006b) (see Table 2.1, below).

Case study

Molly and her husband Frank

Molly (85) has been married to Frank for 58 years; Frank describes Molly as the love of his life and his childhood sweetheart. They have no children of their own but have a niece and nephew, both of whom live some distance away and only manage to see Frank and Molly at Christmas. Your mentor undertook an initial assessment and found that Molly and Frank live in a three-bedroom detached house in a quiet cul-de-sac. They have lived there for 15 years; they have supportive neighbours and a good group of friends who live locally. You have gone to the notes and found that, until recently, they were living independently with no professional help or services.

Molly takes medication for her high blood pressure. She had come into hospital via the emergency department after a fall at home and was admitted due to her breathlessness and the need to find a reason for her fall. Whilst Molly has been on the ward she has undergone a number of tests and has felt very unwell, spending most of her time lying in bed. Occasionally she got out of bed with assistance and sat in a chair supported by pillows.

With your mentor's support you undertake Molly's routine observations (temperature, pulse, respiration and blood pressure) and you also check her fluid balance chart. You find that Molly's temperature is 37.5°C, her pulse is 90 beats/minute and her respirations are 28 per minute. Molly's blood pressure is 98 mmHg diastolic and 140 mmHg systolic. Her fluid intake in the last 24 hours has been 500 ml. Your mentor explains this could indicate Molly has an infection but a dipstick test of her urine did not show any significant abnormalities, although the urine was dark-coloured. Molly has also not been coughing up any sputum. Your mentor informs you and Molly that the results of X-ray examinations, midstream urine sample and blood tests should be available later today. In the meantime you need to keep Molly comfortable and encourage her to drink.

When Frank visits later that morning, you and Molly explain what has happened so far and that the test results should be available later today. Frank explains to you that he is concerned because Molly has lost weight and not eaten anything since coming into hospital and has only had small amounts of water to drink.

Activity 2.1 — *Critical thinking*

Molly is staying in bed for the morning and you have been asked, with a healthcare support worker, to assist Molly with a wash.

- Make notes on what you would be observing when undertaking this task.
- What information given by your mentor helps you decide how you should demonstrate care and compassion and maintain Molly's dignity during this care?
- How would you introduce yourself to Molly?

An outline answer is provided at the end of the chapter.

In Activity 2.1 you could have identified observing Molly's skin, which may give you information about her level of hydration, her oxygen level, skin integrity and previous falls. Observing Molly's breathing could give you clues as to whether she has a chest infection or asthma. Molly's expression could give you lots of information about how she is feeling at the moment; whether she appears relaxed and smiling or in pain. Any interaction with patients can form part of your assessment of their care needs which you can then discuss with your mentor to plan their care.

You may have suggested you could demonstrate care and compassion by introducing yourself, asking whether now is a good time and if she is happy for you to help her. You may also have considered your tone, such as using a warm and friendly voice and non-verbal communication such as smiling and touching her gently on the arm to attract and maintain her attention. We will explore this more later but first we need to determine what the terms care, compassion and communication mean, as these form the first essential care cluster that we will discuss.

Care, compassion and communication

> *The essence of nursing care for older people is about getting to know and value people as individuals through effective assessment, finding out how they want to be cared for from their perspective, and providing care which ensures that respect, dignity and fairness are maintained.*
> (Nursing and Midwifery Council, 2009, p. 3)

Similarly, compassion requires ensuring respect and that any interventions provided protect and maintain dignity, whether they are pain relief, food, dressing or elements of the environment. Compassion is also recognised through kindness and giving thought to the person's emotional and spiritual needs (NHS Confederation, 2012). Jane Cummings, Chief Nursing Officer (2012), in a vision for the future of nurses and the development of the culture of compassionate care, stated that compassion is how care is given through relationships based on empathy, kindness, respect and dignity. To provide compassionate care communication is crucial and it is essential that we as nurses and those we care for can communicate with each other effectively (Department of Health, 2010c).

> *Communication is a process that involves a meaningful exchange between at least two people to convey facts, needs, opinions, thoughts, feelings or other information through both verbal and nonverbal means, including face to face exchanges and the written word.*
> (Department of Health, 2010c)

Care

Simone Roach in the 1980s (cited by Barker, 2011) identified that caring is not unique to nursing but is unique within nursing. She conceptualises caring in her 'five Cs': compassion, competence, confidence, conscience and commitment. Caring is an essential feature of human beings and it is a shared experience between carer and cared for. Nursing theory of the 1970s, 1980s and 1990s recognised the centrality of the relationship between care giver and receiver, highlighting an overarching acceptance of humanistic theory in caring (Barker, 2011). This can also be seen in the work with older people with dementia undertaken by Kitwood (1993) and in the contemporary model of humanisation by Todres et al. (2009). Nursing care can be seen as the way in which we as nurses use our hearts, hands and minds to help people return to health, maintain a sense of well-being or have a 'good death'.

Compassion

A Dignified Revolution, a voluntary movement set up to promote and improve care for older people in hospitals in the UK, urges healthcare professionals, including nurses, to reflect on the following Mumbai hospital motto, adapted from a quotation from Mahatma Gandhi:

> *A patient is the most important person in our hospital. He is not an interruption to our work; he is the purpose of it. He is not an outsider in our hospital; he is a part of it. We are not doing a favour by serving him; he is doing us a favour by giving us an opportunity to do so.*

There has been a lot of discussion in the media about the lack of care, compassion and dignity shown in hospitals in the UK to older people, which could be quite demoralising for you as you start your nursing career (Patients Association, 2009, 2011a, b; *Guardian*, 2011; *Independent*, 2011). There have also been government inquiries into the issue. The Francis Report (2013) identified shortcomings in care, highlighting that there was a focus on meeting targets and getting the job done, without responding to the basic needs of the individual. The Care Quality Commission (2011) stated that 'care' often seems to be broken down into tasks to be completed, focusing on the unit of work, rather than the person, and that kindness and compassion cost nothing.

Behaving towards patients as if they are a task that needs completing is dehumanising, leading to passivity of patients and them viewing themselves as undeserving, reducing their self-respect and possibly leading to poor emotional well-being (Todres et al., 2009). An example which highlights how simple it is to show compassionate care could be you assisting a person with personal hygiene. Simple strategies such as you facilitating choice over the temperature of the water and wash area can promote autonomy and ensure the comfort of the person (D'Hondt et al., 2011). Supporting older people to maintain their personal hygiene is also an excellent opportunity to assess skin integrity, bodily functions and variations in physical stamina (as seen in Activity 2.1) in a more natural and humanised way (Todres et al., 2009). Bowers (2009) emphasises that students must not underestimate the value of giving personal care, both in terms of providing quality care to the patient as well as learning for the student.

There are constant challenges in nursing due to the complexity and rapid pace of healthcare delivery (Bridges et al., 2009) and some suggest this interferes with the ability of nurses to provide compassionate care (Bridges et al., 2009). However, Pearcey (2010) suggests that, whilst it may be more of a challenge doing something in a caring way, it does not necessarily take more time. Pearcey (2010) found that, when observations were being carried out, there was minimal interaction with patients. As an example, when undertaking regular observations you could discuss with patients how they are feeling, their pain and concerns. Compassionate care will be referred to throughout the rest of this chapter as it is crucial in the provision of a humanised approach.

Communication

Communication is at the heart of any nursing practice. The ESCs (Nursing and Midwifery Council, 2010) identify specific areas that need to be demonstrated and achieved during the nursing programme. It is expected that, when you are working with groups or individuals, you will facilitate communication, regardless of whether hearing, vision or speech is compromised, and interact with the person in a manner that is interpreted as warm, sensitive, kind and compassionate, making appropriate use of touch. Also you will listen to, watch for, and respond to verbal and non-verbal cues (Nursing and Midwifery Council, 2010). Within nursing, communication is also conducted through report writing, care planning, incident reporting and record keeping. It is extremely important that these are accurately recorded to reduce any risk of misunderstanding or of inappropriate care.

Communication skills with older people have to address the NMC competencies, acknowledging that many older adults have some loss of vision and hearing. Moriarty et al. (2010) also highlight that individuals may have communication difficulties, such as those arising from conditions like dementia or Parkinson's disease, or following a stroke. Effective communication is more than a means of delivering quality, patient-centred care. It is also the vehicle through which patients' involvement is optimised. Communication is therapeutic and building relationships is the cornerstone of nursing work (Collins, 2009). This has particular relevance to your care of older people, who may not always be able to communicate all their needs due to physical or mental, or even both, levels of impairment. In Activity 2.2 we revisit the case study of Frank and Molly.

Activity 2.2 — ***Critical thinking***

Before you undertake assisting Molly with her personal hygiene you discuss with the healthcare assistant how you will approach communicating with Molly. Make a note of what strategies you both will employ.

An outline answer is provided at the end of the chapter.

When undertaking Activity 2.2 you will probably have identified both verbal and non-verbal types of communication in direct interactions with Molly but also the importance of accurate reporting and collaborative care planning.

How can nurses increase compassionate care?

All the terms used so far related to compassionate care, such as kindness and respect, are difficult to assess quantitatively or objectively, therefore as nurses we need to seek understanding of if and how this occurs by asking the people who are receiving the care.

Bridges et al.'s (2010) systematic review identified that older people and their relatives wanted hospital staff to focus on the following:

- Maintaining identity: See who I am. This was found to be particularly relevant for any hospital admission and loss of identity.
- Creating community: Connect with me.
- Sharing decision making: Involve me.

There are a number of initiatives that support nurses to see patients, connect with them and involve them. The *This is me* leaflet was designed for use with patients who have dementia and are going into hospital, and is considered life-story work (see Useful websites, below).

McKeown et al. (2010) acknowledge that using life-story work with people with dementia enhances person-centred care and reinforces the identity of the person. It also has the additional benefit of facilitating interaction and building relationships (McKeown et al., 2010).

Nolan et al. (2006b) discussed the senses framework as a potential framework for practice which can be seen as addressing the 'see the person, connect with the person and involve the person' wishes of older people. It identified the need to address six senses and can be used alongside Kitwood's (1993) person-centred care for people with dementia and Todres et al.'s (2009) humanising care approaches. These senses were labelled security, belonging, continuity, purpose, achievement and significance, and are described in Table 2.1.

Sense	Achieved by
Security	Provision of regular, clear information
	Access to 'experts' such as medical consultants and clinical nurse specialists
	Regularly asking the older person how he or she feels
	Risk assessment in negotiation with the older person
	Support after discharge, e.g. telephone calls, discharge support
	Staff being aware of the person's life story
	Effective communication
Belonging	Staff using the person's preferred name
	Recognition of importance of relationships with other patients
	Families encouraged to participate in care
	Having designated members of staff to coordinate care
	Flexible visiting times
	Tea and coffee available for patients and visitors
Continuity	Team nursing/named nursing as the system for organising care
	Wards having designated therapy staff
	Access to schemes aimed at enabling an older person to avoid hospital admission unless absolutely necessary, e.g. Rapid Response scheme
	Continuity of support following discharge
	Partnership programmes involving family carers in care giving
	Communication sheets to assist discharge
	Phone calls after discharge and liaison with home care services
	Staff taking time to get to know the older person, perhaps through life history sheets
Purpose	Regular meetings with staff to discuss progress
	Self-medication programmes
	Mutually agreed goals of care
	Being a genuine partner in planning and evaluation

(continued)

Table 2.1 (continued)

Sense	Achieved by
Achievement	Being involved in review of progress and accepting feedback
	Evaluation carried out with the older person
	Care plans and progress sheets accessible
	Promoting independence, mental well-being and motivation
	Multiprofessional approach
Significance	Being involved in care planning and evaluation, e.g. bedside handover
	Biographical assessment
	Resources invested in making the environment comfortable and attractive
	Showing an interest

Table 2.1: The senses framework

Considering Table 2.1, you will be able to identify how you can achieve security, belonging, continuity, purpose, achievement and significance when caring for Molly and Frank. For example, using their preferred names, greeting Frank when he visits and checking if he has any concerns. You could also involve Molly and Frank in your care planning, evaluations and discharge planning.

Nolan et al. (2006b) found that, if placements actively encouraged students to explore the 'person as focus', considering the six senses, then a more holistic view of nursing would be developed. Holistic care is care that incorporates all elements of the person – physical, emotional, social, spiritual and economic. If you see Molly and Frank as people with relationships, families, careers, likes, dislikes and the health problem as just one element of the whole person, it should facilitate your interacting with them as related individuals. It will encourage you to look at all their needs instead of focusing on one area, for example, their need to spend time together or their anxieties about the future.

In all interactions you need to show care and compassion, but there remain tasks that need to be undertaken. Using the ESC of organisational aspects of care, you will be able to explore how you can achieve these in a humanised way in your clinical learning environments.

Organisational aspects of care

Organisational aspects of care identified in the ESCs (Nursing and Midwifery Council, 2010) that nursing students need to achieve are:

- work in partnership with people to make a holistic and systematic assessment of their needs, provide interventions and evaluate their effectiveness;
- develop personalised care plans to promote health and well-being;
- minimise risk; safeguard and protect people from harm;
- respond to feedback;

- ensure continuity when care is transferred;
- be an autonomous and confident member of the multidisciplinary team;
- inspire confidence in others;
- safely delegate and be delegated to, lead, coordinate and manage care;
- work safely under pressure, enhance safety of others and manage risk;
- prevent and manage conflict;
- select and manage medical devices.

You will need to use all of these skills when working with people like Molly and Frank to ensure they receive a quality care experience. We have already identified that to provide care and compassion you need to offer respect and kindness, listen and observe. These skills provide the basis of your organisational skills as well and alongside these your accurate recording and care planning. You can observe your mentor to learn how to respond to feedback, behave within the multidisciplinary team and inspire others. Policies and procedures can be used to develop your understanding of safe use of medical device and safeguarding issues. For example, when you were measuring Molly's regular observations your mentor will have shown you what to do, explained where the policies and procedures for these clinical tasks can be found and then supervised your undertaking them. Whilst undertaking these observations you will have sought Molly's consent, explaining what you were going to do and why. This will support you selecting and managing the medical devices, being delegated to, forming part of your holistic assessment and supporting your working in partnership.

Older people identify that a 'good nurse' has both psychosocial and technical skills (Van der Elst et al., 2012), for example, that the nurse is able not only to undertake technical tasks such as medication administration but also to communicate effectively. Psychosocial skills include good communication and treating people as individuals with dignity. Technical skills include knowledge and understanding of patients' health needs and the ability to coordinate care and make them feel safe. These skills also need to be understood and achieved by student nurses to demonstrate competence in the NMC organisational aspects of care.

Activity 2.3 *Critical thinking*

All of the elements identified within the organisational aspects of care ESCs refer to actions:

- What psychosocial care skills might you need to care for Molly?
- What technical skills might you need to care for Molly?
- What coordination skills might you need to care for Molly?

An outline answer is provided at the end of the chapter.

Assessment is the first stage of the nursing process and as part of your organisational care underpins a number of these essential skills (numbers 9, 10 and 20 of the ESCs). Assessment involves collecting data from a variety of sources. A variety of assessment models are used in clinical settings but all enable the nurse to document and plan care that is appropriate to the individual patient (Taylor et al., 2011). It is about concentrating on what is important to the individual whilst identifying risks and inabilities (Nursing and Midwifery Council, 2009). It is also important to establish a baseline and identify where there is the need to refer to other professionals. Assessment will be discussed further in Chapter 5.

Read the scenario of Martin Ward and consider how he was using his organisational skills.

Scenario: Martin Ward

Martin is a third-year student nurse on a placement with the community nurse, based in a GP surgery. Martin and his mentor, Clare, have been asked to visit Mrs Brown who has recently been discharged from a large acute hospital after a cataract operation on her eye. They have been asked to visit as Mrs Brown lives alone. Clare and Martin discussed Mrs Brown's operation and agreed that Martin should take the lead in assessing Mrs Brown's health needs. On arriving at Mrs Brown's house they knocked at the door and Mrs Brown answered; she appeared a little anxious but after Martin and Clare explained who they were, showed her their identification badges and explained why they were there, she let them into her sitting room.

Martin started by asking Mrs Brown what she would like to be called and she asked them to call her Nora. He then asked Nora how things had been since leaving hospital. Nora explained she had been having problem breathing, and had felt dizzy and nauseous. Martin showed concern and asked if he could undertake a few tests to start with, to assess what was wrong. Nora agreed and Martin took her temperature, pulse, blood pressure and respiration rate. He found her temperature was normal, but her breathing rate, pulse and blood pressure were raised. Martin talked to Nora whilst undertaking these observations, explaining what he was doing and what he had found. During this conversation Nora confided how frightened she had been on returning home, which had led to her not sleeping well and losing her usually good appetite. Martin was also able to ascertain that she did not want to be on her own; she was lonely.

Martin asked Clare if she would contact the GP and inform them of what they had found. He reassured Nora that what she was experiencing was probably due to anxiety but it was best to get the GP to check. He also asked if there was anyone Nora would like him to contact who might be able to spend some time with her. Nora gave him the telephone number of her daughter who lived some distance away. Martin telephoned Nora's daughter whilst Nora sat beside him and her daughter said she would visit her mother the next day and take her mother to see the GP. Nora said she felt this was a good plan and that she would be happy to stay at home by herself knowing her daughter would be there the following day. She thanked Martin for his help. When they had left Nora's house, Clare gave Martin feedback on his interactions. She highlighted how his approach was compassionate and kind and he had managed the risks well.

Activity 2.4

Consider the scenario of Martin Ward. What organisational skills do you think he was using in the scenario?

An outline answer is provided at the end of the chapter.

In Activity 2.4 you may have identified that Martin was able to demonstrate a number of organisational skills in this scenario to his mentor, including delegation (ESC 15), personalised care planning (ESC 9) and risk minimisation (ESCs 9, 18). Martin was assessing Nora's health and well-being by recognising that her experiences may be due to mental or physical problems and he sought to address both.

Despite the wide range of organisational skills in which nurses are expected to demonstrate competence to register with the NMC, it can be seen in the Martin Ward scenario that a number of these skills can be demonstrated in one brief engagement with an older person. In whatever environment you care for older people, you will need to use your organisational skills and be 'the good nurse'.

The next area to be considered in this chapter is the ESC labelled infection control.

Infection prevention and control

Infection control is seen as a significant world health issue, with the World Health Organization (2013a) providing a lead in the promotion of the International Health Regulations (World Health Organization, 2008). In recent years we have seen a number of deaths due to infectious diseases such as avian influenza, methicillin-resistant *Staphylococcus aurea* (MRSA) and *Clostridium difficile.* Older people have reduced immune efficiency, making them more susceptible to bacterial and viral infections (Branning, 2011; Goldstein, 2012), autoimmune and inflammatory pathologies, along with benign and malignant tumours. Therefore this is an important area to consider for this age group. The essential skills for nurses in the infection prevention and control ESC include:

- identification and effective measures to prevent and control infection using local and national policies;
- apply and adapt these to the needs and limitations of all environments;
- effective nursing interventions when someone has an infectious disease;
- comply with hygiene, uniform and dress codes;
- safely and competently apply aseptic principles;
- reduce risks in a variety of settings when handling waste including sharps, linen, bodily products (Nursing and Midwifery Council, 2010).

Scenario: Megan Blackmore, part 1

Megan is on her first placement in a specialist dementia nursing home and her mentor, Susan, has recently undertaken the mentorship programme; Susan is very enthusiastic and hopes to be a good role model for Megan. Megan is very keen but has limited care experience.

Susan explains to Megan the expectations related to uniform, attendance, fire and emergency exits on their first meeting. She also shows Megan how to access all the policies and procedures for the unit and

(continued)

continued ...

tells Megan that if she has any queries, she should just ask her. Susan explains that the most important thing for Megan to understand is that, for all the people that live there, it is their home. Susan explains she needs to do a dressing on one of the resident's leg ulcers and Megan is keen to get involved. Susan checks the equipment she needs in the clinic room and then seeks out the woman, whose name is Gladys, to ask if she would like the dressing done in her room or the clinic. Gladys does not express a preference so it is decided to do it in the clinic room where infection risks can be minimised.

Activity 2.5 — *Critical thinking*

What do Susan and Megan need to consider to control the risk of infection for Gladys?

An outline answer is provided at the end of the chapter.

As you will have identified in Activity 2.5, Susan and Megan will have had to consider a large number of potential areas of risk: risks associated with the environment (the clinic room), risks associated with the wound, any potential infections already in the wound and any potential infection that may be introduced. For example, does Gladys have any previous and current medical history? What is her nutritional state and does she have any current infections, such as MRSA? As we know, Gladys has dementia so Susan and Megan will need to consider carefully how they explain what is happening and why; see scenario part 2, below.

Gladys has the most common type of ulcer, which is a venous leg ulcer. These occur more frequently in older people, mostly women, and treatment usually involves compression bandaging, elevation and activity. Leg ulcers are at risk of becoming infected, leading to significant health implications such as blood poisoning. Susan explains to Megan that, due to Gladys's dementia, she forgets why she is wearing compression bandages and usually take them off after a while as they are not comfortable, increasing the risk of spreading infection. Gladys also is not keen on elevating her leg to relieve the pressure. Ensuring she has regular exercise is not a problem as Gladys enjoys walking around the home saying hello to everyone.

Scenario: Megan Blackmore, part 2

Megan observed Susan's interactions with Gladys. Susan used short sentences that were clear and without any medical jargon to explain to Gladys that her leg ulcer needed a new dressing. She also introduced Megan and explained that Megan is a student nurse and needed to learn how to do dressings and asked if it would be all right if Megan watched her change the dressing. Gladys looked unsure at Megan but when Megan smiled at her she agreed.

Susan and Megan had already laid out all the equipment they needed in the clinic room and had wiped down the surfaces and the trolley for the dressing pack with alcohol gel. Gladys was made comfortable in a chair with her leg on a stool that had been covered with a sterilised towel. Susan calmly and gently explained what she was going to do, again checking Gladys understood. She then explained she needed to take off the old dressing and check her leg. Susan asked Gladys if she would like to listen to some music whilst she changed the dressing. Gladys enjoyed music and readily agreed; Susan turned on Classic FM on the radio.

Susan explained to Gladys and Megan what she was doing as she undertook the task; she explained that she and Megan needed to put on gloves and aprons so that she did not get any infection in Gladys's ulcer, whilst Gladys watched them. The wound seemed to cause minimal pain for Gladys but every time there was a risk of discomfort Susan stopped and explained what was going to happen, including removing the old dressing and cleaning the ulcerated site. At the end Gladys was thanked for being patient and allowing Megan to watch and asked if Megan could do the dressing next time. Gladys agreed. Afterwards Susan explained to Megan that she had used aseptic technique and had a discussion with her about what this meant.

Whilst Susan needed to reduce any risk of infection for Gladys or from Gladys infecting other residents, she also needed to work in a psychologically therapeutic manner given Gladys's cognitive impairment. Given the frequently complex presentation of older people, undertaking what might be considered routine clinical activities is more challenging. As you could see from Megan's scenario, she was developing not only infection control skills and wound management skills but also advanced communication skills.

This section has considered the ESC of infection prevention and control; these are important skills whatever environment you work in. The policies and procedures will differ depending on the environment but it is even more important when working with older people due to their greater susceptibility to infection (Branning, 2011; Goldstein, 2012).

A person's ability to withstand infection is significantly influenced by nutrition and hydration and this is the next ESC to be explored.

Nutrition and fluid management

Age Concern first evidenced concerns about the malnutrition of older people in hospital in its report, *Hungry to be Heard* (2006). Sadly, this was not a new problem as the Department of Health Essence of Care, developed in 2001, was created due to reports of poor basic nursing care, including nutrition (Department of Health, 2001a); this was updated in 2010 (Department of Health, 2010c). Age UK provided a follow-up report, *Still Hungry to be Heard* (Age UK, 2010), showing that little improvement had been made and that around 175,000 patients enter hospital malnourished and 185,000 leave malnourished. The report also stated that nurses do not ensure vulnerable patients receive the help they need to prevent malnutrition. The recent Francis Report (2013) again highlights the continued occurrence and consequences of poor nutrition and fluids.

Nutrition and fluid management are essential for life and as nurses we need to ensure that those we care for have adequate food and fluids. The ESC for nutrition and fluid management (Nursing and Midwifery Council, 2010) states that nurses need to be able to:

- assist choice in the provision of adequate nutritional and fluid diets;
- monitor nutritional and fluid status and formulate care plan;
- create a conducive environment;
- support those unable to receive food by mouth or fluids independently.

The NHS (NHS Choices, 2013) advises that everyone has a healthy balanced diet, which includes:

- plenty of fruit and vegetables – aim for at least five portions of a variety of fruit and veg a day;
- plenty of bread, rice, potatoes, pasta and other starchy foods – choose wholegrain varieties if you can;
- some milk and dairy foods;
- some meat, fish, eggs, beans and other non-dairy sources of protein – try to eat at least two portions of fish a week, including a portion of oily fish;
- just a small amount of foods and drinks that are high in fat or sugar.

For people over 60 they recommend eating fibre-rich foods such as wholegrain cereals and bread to reduce the higher risks of constipation and digestive problems in this age group. It is also important to maintain iron intake as low iron will reduce energy levels, but not to eat over 70 grams of red meat a day. Iron can be found in red meats, oily fish, beans and pulses or fortified breakfast cereals. Older people, particularly women, are at risk of osteoporosis so it is important to ensure they eat calcium-rich foods such as dairy product. Dairy products that are low in fat can now be bought easily. It is also important that vitamins and minerals are kept within the guidelines; for example, an older person is more at risk of high blood pressure and taking over 6 grams of salt a day will increase this risk. Likewise, too much vitamin A, which is high in liver, may increase the risk of bone fractures.

Remaining hydrated is even more important as dehydration can quickly lead to significant health problems such as infections and confusion. An older person should drink about 1.2 litres of fluid a day and if the weather is warm or the person is exercising this will need to be increased.

Activity 2.6 *Critical thinking*

Frank is concerned Molly is losing weight and from the information you have you can see she is not drinking enough. What will you do to address Molly's eating and drinking?

An outline answer is provided at the end of the chapter.

In Activity 2.6 you probably recognised a number of methods for assessing and improving Molly's nutritional and fluid status. The first step may have been to have a conversation with Molly and Frank together to explore the concerns and what you can all do together to improve Molly's diet. These will have included checking what she liked to eat and drink, whether she has any swallowing difficulties, spending time with her to ensure she could access food and drink and whether she needs any additional equipment. You will also probably have identified organisational skills such as recording what she ate and drank, how much and when. You may have considered infection prevention and control skills as well.

Food and fluid are essential for life. It is therefore imperative that nurses develop the skills to manage nutrition and fluids. When working with older people with multiple diagnoses, higher vulnerability and possible cognitive impairment, you need to be particularly alert to these needs. Undertaking practice placements with older people can enhance awareness and skills in this area. Risk and assessment of nutrition and fluid needs will be further explored in Chapter 5.

Medication managment

The final ESC to be considered in this chapter is medicine management. You must develop your knowledge and skills in this area to ensure safe and effective practice. The ESC for medication management states you need to:

- correctly and safely undertake medicine calculation, working within the legal and ethical framework underpinning safe and effective medicine management;
- have a comprehensive knowledge of medicines, their actions, risks and benefits, their supply and administration to individuals and via group direction;
- safely order, receive, store and dispose of medicines in any setting;
- administer in a safe and timely manner working in partnership with patients and carers;
- keep accurate records;
- evaluate up-to-date information, working within national and local policy guidelines.

Keenan et al. (2011) identified the increased risk factor for older people as they are more likely to be on multiple medications, known as polypharmacy. Polypharmacy is prevalent in older people and is a known risk factor for morbidity and mortality (Hajjar et al., 2007). This means that when administering medication to older people you need to monitor them more closely and have a detailed understanding of the medication they are receiving, including their action, adverse effects and potential interactions (Kaufman, 2011).

Case study: Brenda Boyle

Brenda is currently having respite care in a local nursing home so that her daughter can take a holiday with her family. Brenda has a number of health problems: she has type 2 diabetes, high cholesterol, temporal arteritis, chronic renal failure and vascular dementia. She has had two pulmonary embolisms and two minor strokes. At home her medication and associated blood tests have been quite stable. She is taking:

- *metformin 500 mg three times a day with breakfast, lunch and evening meal for her diabetes;*
- *warfarin 3 mg once a day;*
- *simvastatin 40 mg once a day;*
- *prednisolone 10 mg four times a day (Table 2.2).*

(continued)

continued ...

Medication	Therapeutic effect	Adverse effects	Lifestyle implications
Metformin	It is a diabetic drug that helps control blood sugar. Increased blood sugar can lead to heart disease, stroke, nerve damage, retinopathy, kidney disease	Seek medical advice if: muscle weakness, numb or cold feeling in arms or legs, trouble breathing, feeling dizzy, stomach pain, vomiting, slow or uneven heart rate, rapid weight gain, fever, chills	To improve well-being with diabetes: Eat a healthy diet, high in fibre, fruit and vegetables, low in fat, sugar and salt. Take regular exercise. Do not smoke, limit alcohol. Blood tests to check blood sugar
Warfarin	An anticoagulant; it reduces the formation of thrombi, which can block blood vessels, leading to problems such as strokes, pulmonary embolism or deep-vein thrombosis	Blood in urine, black faeces, severe bruising, bleeding gums, blood in vomit, unusual headaches. Do not take aspirin or ibuprofen with this drug. Everything ingested can have an impact on warfarin levels	Regular blood test to check level Limit alcohol Regular balanced diet Avoid cranberry juice
Simvastatin	Reduce cholesterol in the blood. High cholesterol can lead to plaques in the blood vessels which stop the blood reaching the organs, causing cell death	Muscle problems, memory problems, fever, vomiting, headaches, constipation, hair loss, indigestion, liver problems. Interactions can occur with warfarin	Limit alcohol Low-fat diet Avoid grapefruit juice
Prednisolone	A steroid; it has been prescribed to treat temporal arteritis to reduce inflammation and pain	Psychological: depressed, anxious, confused, mood changes, hallucinations. Weight gain, weakening of bones, increased blood pressure, stomach ulcers, increased risk of infection. Risk of developing diabetes, high blood pressure and osteoporosis	Balanced healthy diet Reduce risk of infection

Table 2.2: Brenda's medications

As with Brenda Boyle, many older people have complex health needs and polypharmacy. Many drugs interact with each other and with lifestyle issues, such as exercise, food and fluid intake. Considering the case study of Brenda, undertake Activity 2.7.

Activity 2.7 — *Critical thinking*

What factors will you need to consider in relation to managing Brenda's medication whilst she is in the nursing home?

An outline answer is provided at the end of the chapter.

In the case study of Brenda you can see that, to maintain her health, Brenda takes a number of medications, all of which have side-effect profiles, and will also be affected by lifestyle factors such as diet, amount of fluid intake and exercise. Brenda's preferences for how she takes the medications, with which foods and at what time of day will need to be considered. Because of her physical incapacity she may require medications to be in fluid formulations or given to her in special containers. If guidelines are not followed Brenda's health will be at risk. The nurse's responsibility is also to ensure that medications are ordered, stored and administered in accordance with local policy and the pharmaceutical manufacturer's recommendations.

Whilst you are on placements you will be able to observe how medications are managed in a variety of settings. You will also observe how medications are administered and how any individual needs are catered for, in particular if a person is elderly, anxious or forgetful. You will gain knowledge of medications, their uses and administration in the university lectures. The guidance and support from mentors in practice placements will help you by explaining the guidelines, recognising the relevance of these to each individual older person's needs. This will be further discussed in Chapter 5.

Chapter summary

The Department of Health and NHS Commissioning Board (2012) identify that being a nurse is an amazing role and that we support people and their families when they are most vulnerable. Keenan et al. (2011) acknowledge that working with older people requires complex skills which are sometimes not always recognised. This chapter has aimed to identify some of the learning opportunities that can be gained through working with older people. By linking activities to case studies and scenarios it has facilitated reflection on potential learning and demonstration of achieving competence in practice. This is not an exhaustive list but highlights some of the issues in each of the ESCs (compassionate care and communication; organisational aspects of care; infection prevention and control; nutrition and fluids; medication management) and the need to reflect continuously on practice to learn and develop.

Activities: brief outline answers

Activity 2.1

Suggested responses: this list is not exhaustive.

Observations

- Skin: colour (bruising, bluish), dry, flaky, clammy, loose (weight loss), temperature, warm, cold;
- Facial expression: upset, calm, relaxed, in pain, frightened;
- Movements: does this cause pain, is it restricted, muscle tone;
- Smell: stale urine, pear drops, alcohol;
- Communication: is she able to talk easily, or does she find it difficult to find words. Is she confused?

Compassionate care Curtains or door closed; signs to ensure privacy; do not disturb; talk to Molly directly; have a calm manner and approach; appear not to rush; give Molly time; allow Molly to participate as much as she is able; communication skills; reassurance; empathy; sensitivity; comfort; warmth; introducing yourself; whether now is a good time; happy to help; talk to Molly about her interests, her likes and dislikes.

Introduction Explain who you are and what your role is using a friendly, warm tone. Ask her what name she would like you to call her and how she is feeling.

Activity 2.2

You may have discussed who was going to take the lead and who would say what. You may need to consider:

- Verbal communication: tone; pitch; rate and volume;
- Non-verbal communication: eye contact; use of touch; professional appearance; organised, collecting everything you need; avoid leaving during the personal care giving;
- Proxemics: personal space; distance;
- Documentation, such as handover, record keeping, nursing notes, interprofessional notes, discuss plan.

Activity 2.3

Suggested responses: this list is not exhaustive.

- Psychosocial care skills: building a relationship, developing rapport through communication – listening, reflecting, giving feedback;
- Technical skills: taking measurements, for example, blood pressure, temperature, giving medication, using the computer, record keeping;
- Coordination skills: care planning, making referrals to other professionals.

Activity 2.4

Delegation; personalised care planning; risk assessment and management; holistic assessment.

Activity 2.5

Room; patient's current health status; factors that will impact, such as nutritional status, medication. Past medical history, such as previous infections; condition of the wound; redness, swelling; general observations; aseptic technique; general environment; equipment; protective clothing; hand washing.

Activity 2.6

Suggested responses: this list is not exhaustive.

Ensure choice and knowledge of food preferences; monitoring food and fluid intake; assistance, which could be positioning; assistance to eat; adaptations, e.g. cutlery and equipment; clear documentation and charting; weight monitoring; use of body mass index; use of nutritional assessment tools such as the Malnutrition Universal Screening Tool (MUST) scale.

Involvement of dietician for advice and support; physiotherapist to help in positioning and comfort; occupational therapist for equipment and support; doctors to review medication; care staff to be aware of the importance of ensuring nutritional requirement and documentation; reassessment and evaluation.

Activity 2.7

What time of day did she have her meals and what were her portion sizes?

Ensure dietary requirements are met; adequate intake; low sugar; low fat; check what foods must be avoided for possible interactions, e.g. grapefruit juice and warfarin.

Ensure plenty of fluids, particularly water due to medication and chronic renal failure.

Skin observation: check for bruising; awareness of any abnormal bleeding (warfarin and prednisolone).

Importance of exercise, maintaining mobility (reducing risk of further embolisms); checking ankle or calf swelling.

Importance of infection control.

Useful websites

http://www.alzheimers.org.uk/site/scripts/documents_info.php?documentID=1290

Access the *This is me* leaflet and make notes on how the information would have helped in your assessment and care for Molly.

BAPEN: **http://www.bapen.org.uk**

http://dignifiedrevolution.org.uk/news/34-compassion/436-the-point-of-care-enabling-compassionate-care-in-acute-hospital-settings.html

Royal College of Nursing: http://nursingstandard.rcnpublishing.co.uk/shared/media/pdfs/CaringForOlderPeople.pdf

Social Care Institute for Excellence: http://www.scie.org.uk/adults/safeguarding/index.asp

http://www.youtube.com/watch?v=MTcopj6dYWQ

Watch the scenario called 'This is me'. Compare your previous notes on how you would provide compassionate care to the nurses shown on the clip.

The clip showed care that was uncaring, uncompassionate and devoid of dignity. It reinforces some of the current reports regarding patients' experiences.

Further reading

Firth-Cozens, J and Cornwell, J (2009) *The Point of Care: Enabling compassionate care in acute hospital settings.* London: Kings Fund.

Patients Association (2009) *Patients ... Not Numbers, People ... Not Statistics.* London: Patients Association. Available from: **http://www.patients-association.com/Portals/0/Public/Files/Research%20Publications/Patients%20not%20numbers,%20people%20not%20statistics.pdf**

Chapter 3
Vulnerability and old age

Vanessa Heaslip

NMC Standards for Pre-registration Nursing Education

Domain 1: Professional values

2. All nurses must practise in a holistic, non-judgmental, caring and sensitive manner that avoids assumptions, supports social inclusion; recognises and respects individual choice; and acknowledges diversity. Where necessary, they must challenge inequality, discrimination and exclusion from access to care.
4. All nurses must work in partnership with service users, carers, families, groups, communities and organisations. They must manage risk, and promote health and wellbeing while aiming to empower choices that promote self-care and safety.

Domain 2: Communication and interpersonal skills

1. All nurses must build partnerships and therapeutic relationships through safe, effective and non-discriminatory communication. They must take account of individual differences, capabilities and needs.
2. All nurses must use a range of communication skills and technologies to support person-centred care and enhance quality and safety. They must ensure people receive all the information they need in a language and manner that allows them to make informed choices and share decision making. They must recognise when language interpretation or other communication support is needed and know how to obtain it.

Domain 3: Nursing practice and decision making

9. All nurses must be able to recognise when a person is at risk and in need of extra support and protection and take reasonable steps to protect them from abuse.

Domain 4: Leadership, management and team working

1. All nurses must act as change agents and provide leadership through quality improvement and service development to enhance people's wellbeing and experiences of healthcare.
4. All nurses must be self-aware and recognise how their own values, principles and assumptions may affect their practice. They must maintain their own personal and professional development, learning from experience, through supervision, feedback, reflection and evaluation.

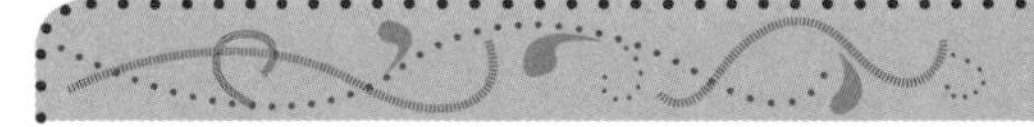

NMC Essential Skills Clusters (ESCs)

This chapter will support the following ESCs:

Cluster: Care, compassion and communication

2. People can trust the newly registered graduate nurse to engage in person centred care empowering people to make choices about how their needs are met when they are unable to meet them themselves.
3. People can trust the newly registered graduate nurse to respect them as individuals and strive to help them preserve their dignity at all times.
4. People can trust a newly qualified graduate nurse to engage with them and their family or carers within their cultural environments in an acceptant and anti-discriminatory manner free from harassment and exploitation.
5. People can trust the newly registered graduate nurse to engage with them in a warm, sensitive and compassionate way.

Organisational aspects of care

9. People can trust the newly registered graduate nurse to treat them as partners and work with them to make a holistic and systematic assessment of their needs; to develop a personalised plan that is based on mutual understanding and respect for their individual situation promoting health and well-being, minimising risk of harm and promoting their safety at all times.
11. People can trust the newly registered graduate nurse to safeguard children and adults from vulnerable situations and support and protect them from harm.

Chapter aims

By the end of this chapter you will be able to:

- discuss vulnerability and its links to nursing older people
  - exploring the etic and emic perspective of vulnerability;
- discuss professional obligations with regard to caring for older people;
- explore how vulnerability relates to safeguarding;
- critically challenge perceptions of older people as a vulnerable group through discussing stereotyping, dehumanising, infantilisation and welfarism;
- recognise that nurses can also experience feeling vulnerable and identifying strategies for dealing with this.

Introduction

Older people are often considered by health and social care practitioners as a vulnerable group. As nurses we need to understand what this means and why this may be so. In this chapter we begin by exploring vulnerability within the context of healthcare, examining why it is important that nurses are aware of the concept of vulnerability. We will revisit Molly and Frank's story from Chapter 2, and consider how and why they may have felt vulnerable. In doing so we will see how nurses can reduce or sometimes even increase a person's experience of vulnerability.

We then go on to examine vulnerability as a mechanism to protect older people from harm in line with adult safeguarding policies. You will be able to critique current policy guidance, examining how a policy which means to protect vulnerable adults could potentially increase their vulnerability through perpetuating the stereotype that older people are frail and require protection.

Last, we look at the vulnerability that nurses feel because of the personal engagement within a therapeutic relationship. You will be able to reflect on and question your own practice and experiences of vulnerability, and identify ways of managing this productively.

Vulnerability and healthcare

In healthcare some groups of individuals are often referred to as vulnerable. Let's start by finding out what we mean by this.

Activity 3.1 *Reflection*

Within the context of your practice you may have heard some groups of patients or service users identified as vulnerable. Or you may yourself think of certain groups of people that you work with are vulnerable. Make a list of these and then write brief notes about what it is about these groups which makes you think that they are vulnerable.

An outline answer is provided at the end of the chapter.

Within this activity you may have identified people who are ill as being potentially vulnerable. Indeed, as nurses we come across vulnerable people every day, as everyone feels vulnerable when their health is compromised. This is compounded when you are in unfamiliar surroundings, situations or relationships (Nursing and Midwifery Council, 2002), such as going into hospital or another healthcare setting. Barker (2005) identifies loss of identity as a major reason why becoming a patient can lead individuals to feeling vulnerable. For example, when people are admitted to hospital they often have to remove their clothes and wear nightwear, they are separated from their loved ones and family and have limited space around them in which to place personal belongings of significance: in essence they lose themselves and become like every other patient. Prolonged feelings of vulnerability are detrimental to both physical and psychological health, because feeling vulnerable can be linked to feelings of helplessness and increased anxiety levels (Rogers, 1997). As such, you need to understand what vulnerability is and how, through your interactions with patients, you can either reduce or increase these feelings of vulnerability.

Some of you may have identified in Activity 3.1 that older people are frequently identified as a vulnerable group in health and social care, but have you ever stopped to consider why this is so? Before continuing to explore why older people may feel vulnerable we need to make sure you have a good understanding of the term itself.

Definitions

Vulnerability is a poorly defined concept in nursing, even though it is often used in healthcare to describe groups of people. Exploring the Latin roots of the term identifies *vuln* (wound) and *vulnare* (to wound), whilst dictionary definitions identify the notion of harm, which could be either physical or psychological, as well as a danger or threat to the person. From these it can be seen that the term vulnerable is essentially linked to wounding, threat or harm of an individual, which could be physical, spiritual, psychological, social, financial or environmental.

It is also important to remember that the degree of vulnerability a person feels is affected by his or her individual perception of the situation. For example, two patients may undergo the same procedure with the same staff in the same general practice surgery, but one may feel more vulnerable than the other. As vulnerability is an individual experience, if patients say they are feeling vulnerable, then they are. Vulnerability is also situational, which means that a person may feel vulnerable in one situation but not another. It is this situational nature of vulnerability which we see in the next part of Molly and Frank's case study.

Case study: Molly and Frank, part 1

Molly (85) and Frank (89) have been married for 58 years; Frank describes Molly as the love of his life. They have no children of their own but have a niece and nephew who both live some distance away and only manage to see Frank and Molly at Christmas. Molly and Frank live in a three-bedroom detached house in a quiet cul-de-sac. They have lived there for 15 years, and regularly speak of how hard they had to work in order to buy the house. Both Molly and Frank are exceptionally happy where they live, as they have supportive neighbours and a good group of local friends. They are living completely independently without any professional help or services. However, recently Molly has needed more help from Frank, especially in climbing the stairs. This had led both of them to consider whether they should move to a bungalow. They are both reluctant to do so as they are very happy where they are living and don't really want to leave their community.

Considering the case study, Molly and Frank may not actually feel vulnerable at all; they are living happily in their own home in a neighbourhood they like. Even though Frank recently has been assisting Molly more, she may feel safe and secure at home with Frank's help and therefore not perceive herself to be vulnerable at all. But circumstances can change.

Case study: Molly and Frank, part 2

In the early hours of the morning Molly fell at home and could not get up as she was feeling very breathless. Frank called the paramedics who came and said that she needed to go to hospital. Molly reluctantly agreed and was taken by the paramedics to the emergency department. Molly underwent a variety of tests, such as X-rays, blood tests and heart monitoring. The blood tests showed that Molly had a high potassium level and so she was admitted to an elderly care ward to investigate this, as well as potential reasons for the fall.

Molly could now feel very vulnerable in this changed situation. As nurses, we may not actually stop to consider how Molly may feel and think about what happened as we are busy treating her. However, without understanding how Molly feels, how can we, as nurses, ensure we meet her needs? Read Molly's account of what happened.

Case study: Molly's story

I woke up and it was dark, I looked at the clock and I saw that it was 2.24 a.m., Frank was fast asleep beside me. I felt incredibly thirsty so had to get up for a drink. I walked down the stairs towards the kitchen. Suddenly I felt myself falling and I shouted. I am lying on the floor and my heart is racing, I see Frank running towards me, asking me if I am OK. Am I? I don't know ... I try to move but I cannot seem to catch my breath. Frank tells me it's OK ... but I must admit I feel kind of scared and shaky.

The next thing I know Frank has opened the door and there are two ambulance men there asking me questions. I try to answer, but I can't, I just feel so breathless. I am worried about Frank as he looks tired and he really needs to be in bed. The paramedics put something in my arm which hurts and tell me and Frank they need to take me to the hospital. Frank looks worried, which worries me. I am scared of what is happening but I don't really want to make a fuss, I wish they would just put me back to bed so Frank can go to sleep.

We go to the emergency department and suddenly I feel invaded, there are nurses and doctors all asking me questions and touching me. I don't really know what they are doing but I am getting more and more worried. What are all these tests for? I don't say anything, I just do as they ask; I mean, they are the experts. I am worried about Frank; I hope he is OK.

Looking at the experience from Molly's perspective it is evident that she is frightened and scared about Frank and about what is happening. She is in a whirlwind, does not really know what is going on and does not feel in control. Molly's experience of acute healthcare is a common one. Sørlie et al. (2006) studied patients' experiences of being cared for in an acute care ward, and vulnerability arose as one of the themes. Patients expressed feelings of helplessness; a fear of what is happening, confusion regarding what is going on around them and an uncertainty of their diagnosis, all of which we can see in Molly's experience. Therefore we can conclude that in this situation Molly is feeling vulnerable: she is unsure what is happening and feels a lack of control. Control is vital to one's experience of vulnerability in that the more control individuals feel they have over a situation, then the less vulnerable they will feel; conversely, the less control they have then the more vulnerable they will feel (Figure 3.1).

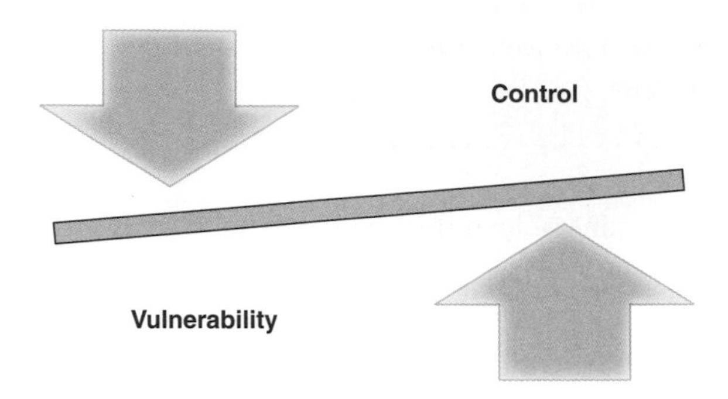

Figure 3.1: Relationship between vulnerability and control

Healthcare practitioners generally view vulnerability as a feature of vulnerable groups, identified by their increased risk of poor health, and who experience higher morbidity (illness) and mortality (death) (Flaskerud and Winslow, 1998). Older people are often seen as a vulnerable group (Spiers, 2000; Rydeman and Törnkvist, 2006) due to this increased likelihood of morbidity and mortality. Stenbock-Hult and Sarvimäki (2011) take a broader perspective, saying that older people are perceived as vulnerable because ageing is categorised by increasing physical, mental and social vulnerability. Lastly, Brocklehurst and Laurenson (2008) think that, whilst people can be vulnerable at any age, many people associate the term with older people. Yet we have to ask whether vulnerability is an inevitable consequence of ageing. We know that ageing is not a homogeneous experience (the same for everyone), but an individual one. Research by Myall et al. (2009) exploring perceived vulnerability on depressive symptoms and perceived general well-being in older people identified that a perception of vulnerability was attenuated in older adults who possessed a strong sense of coherence and positive attitude towards life, thereby identifying that not all older people perceived themselves as vulnerable. These different views can be explored further by considering the etic and emic perspectives of vulnerability.

Etic versus emic perspectives of vulnerability

Spiers (2000, p. 716) conducted a concept analysis and identified two main approaches to viewing vulnerability which she called the 'etic' and 'emic' perspectives (these terms were borrowed from anthropology, in which they are commonly used to explore different ways of understanding human behaviour). The etic or outsider perspective relates to the *susceptibility to and possibility of harm*; it is externally evaluated or judged by others, for example, health and social care practitioners, or society. This approach focuses upon the population of older people and identifies that vulnerability is a dichotomous experience (you are either vulnerable or you are not). Under the etic perspective, all older people would be viewed as vulnerable due to the increased poorer health outcomes, increased financial vulnerability and potential for social isolation mentioned previously.

In contrast, Spiers (2000, p. 716) also recognised an alternative perspective which related to a *state of being threatened and a feeling of fear or harm,* which she called the *emic* or insider perspective. This perspective, rather than assuming all older people are vulnerable, recognises that vulnerability is a subjective, individual experience that can only be identified by the individual actually experiencing it, therefore it is internally judged. From this perspective, vulnerability is exactly what the person experiencing it says it is, recognising that whilst some older people may experience feeling vulnerable, others may not.

In order to illuminate the etic and emic perspectives of vulnerability, read the poem, *Crabbit Old Woman.* The authorship of this famous poem is not clear; however it is thought to have been found in the bedside locker of a patient who had spent some time in a hospital ward.

Crabbit Old Woman

What do you see, what do you see?
Are you thinking, when you look at me
A crabbit old woman, not very wise,
Uncertain of habit, with far-away eyes,
Who dribbles her food and makes no reply
When you say in a loud voice,
I do wish you'd try.
Who seems not to notice the things that you do
And forever is losing a stocking or shoe.
Who, unresisting or not, lets you do as you will
With bathing and feeding the long day is filled.
Is that what you're thinking,
Is that what you see?
Then open your eyes,
Nurse, you're looking at me.
I'll tell you who I am as I sit here so still!
As I rise at your bidding, as I eat at your will.
I'm a small child of 10 with a father and mother,
Brothers and sisters, who loved one another
A young girl of 16 with wings on her feet,
Dreaming that soon now a lover she'll meet,
A bride soon at 20 – my heart gives a leap,
Remembering the vows that I promised to keep.
At 25 now I have young of my own
Who need me to build a secure happy home;
A woman of 30, my young now grow fast,
Bound to each other with ties that should last;
At 40, my young sons have grown and are gone,

But my man's beside me to see I don't mourn;
At 50 once more babies play around my knee,
Again we know children, my loved one and me.
Dark days are upon me, my husband is dead,
I look at the future, I shudder with dread,
For my young are all rearing young of their own.
And I think of the years and the love that I've known;
I'm an old woman now and nature is cruel,
Tis her jest to make old age look like a fool.
The body is crumbled, grace and vigour depart,
There is now a stone where I once had a heart,
But inside this old carcass, a young girl still dwells,
And now and again my battered heart swells,
I remember the joy, I remember the pain,
And I'm loving and living life over again.
I think of the years all too few – gone too fast.
And accept the stark fact that nothing can last,
So open your eyes, nurse, open and see,
Not a crabbit old woman, look closer –
See me.

Activity 3.2 *Critical thinking*

Reread the poem *Crabbit Old Woman* and underline the words and/or lines which depict the etic or external perspective of the patient, and then circle the words and/or lines which depict the emic or lived experience.

An outline answer is provided at the end of the chapter.

Whilst the background of this poem is unclear, some say it was written by a patient and left in a bedside locker whilst others say it was written by a nurse. What it illuminates for me, as a nurse, is the etic and emic perspective of viewing older people. At the start of the poem we see the etic or nurse's view of the person with words such as crabbit, old, not very wise, uncertain of habit, dribbles, losing a stocking or shoe. The image that this evokes is someone who is frail, confused and muddled, who needs assistance with eating and managing activities of daily living. Whereas in contrast, the emic perspective includes words such as my heart gives a leap, wings on her feet, young girl dwells, battered heart swells, remember the joy, remember the pain, loving and living life over again. What these words invoke is someone who has lived a life, vitality and living, so instead of seeing 'a patient' we can see 'a person', illustrating the difference between the external (etic) and internal (emic) views of vulnerability.

This difference in perspectives between nurses and older people has been researched by Abley et al. (2011), who identified that older people viewed vulnerability as an emotional response to being in a specific situation over which they had little or no control, whereas the professionals perceived vulnerability to be linked to risk factors such as being mentally or physically frail and living alone. Thus the professional view focused upon an etic approach to vulnerability and the older people focused upon the emic perspective. Therefore you need to be cautious when working with older people that you focus upon both the etic and emic approaches, otherwise you will fail to address your clients' needs fully, and could instead be inadvertently increasing your clients' vulnerability through discriminatory practices. It is to these practices that we now turn.

Vulnerability and discrimination against older people

Key issues to emerge from research with older people relate to the negative and discriminatory attitudes towards them (Hoban et al., 2011). Particular issues that arose were lack of respect, empathy, listening and compassion. These concerns have also been identified in governmental reports (Francis, 2011; Parliamentary and Health Service Ombudsman, 2011; Commission on Dignity in Care for Older People, 2012). These reports show that there was a negative, neglectful culture within these care settings which had a negative impact upon the quality of care that older people received. In addition, at times, individual staff members provided poor-quality care, which is in contrast to the professional values set out in the Code of Conduct (Nursing and Midwifery Council, 2008b).

The Care and Compassion Report (Parliamentary and Health Service Ombudsman, 2011) included the case of Mr D:

> *Mr D was diagnosed with advanced stomach cancer and was planned to be discharged home. On the day of discharge his family arrives to find him in a distressed condition behind drawn curtains in a chair. He had been waiting several hours to go home. He was in pain, desperate to go to the toilet and unable to ask for help because he was so dehydrated he could not speak properly or swallow. The emergency call bell had been placed beyond his reach. When the family asked for assistance to help him onto the commode he called out in pain.*

Staff were neglectful in their care of Mr D; he was dehydrated and unable to ask for assistance as the call bell was not located within his reach. For us as staff, remembering to ensure that patients have access to the call bell is such a little thing; however, it is easy to see in this scenario that the ramifications of this failure were major. During this episode Mr D must have felt vulnerable, in that he was in physical pain and in no doubt discomfort due to his dehydration. If Mr D was a member of your family, you would not be happy with this experience of care, and this is a benchmark you should use when grading your care.

We must ask ourselves why these experiences of care happen although nurses enter the profession desiring to make a difference. Caring for older people is a Cinderella service which is not perceived within or outside the nursing profession as glamorous and is not well funded. Correspondingly, nurses who work there are often perceived as inferior to those working in other specialities such as critical care or surgery. Alabaster (2007) concurs that caring for older people is seen by some nurses as heavy work, arduous, monotonous and a waste of time, yet older people are by far the largest client group of the NHS because of the ageing population and changing patterns of illness (see Chapters 1 and 2).

In Chapter 6 we explore discrimination and ageism in more depth. However, in order to explore why some older people will feel vulnerable, we need to understand dehumanisation, stereotyping, welfarism and medicalisation, infantilisation and elderspeak, which are all processes of discrimination.

Dehumanisation

This process refers to the ways in which people are stripped of their human attributes and qualities. For example, this can occur during the process of hospitalisation as clients' clothes and personal belongings are removed and they lose their identity and individuality and become patients. Dehumanisation is further perpetuated by the language used in healthcare which refers to people by their condition or attributes, rather than focusing upon their individuality: 'the femur fracture in bed 6' rather than 'John Elliot, retired butcher, and family man'. This is a particular risk when caring for people with dementia, who are less able than others to articulate or present themselves as a person with a past life experience. It is all too easy for such patients to be dehumanised, so instead of seeing a person with a life history, a nurse may just see a task to be undertaken.

In a paper exploring perceptions of dementia, co-written by someone living with dementia (Ann), the author articulates, *dementia is not an identity, it is a label* (Sabat et al., 2011, p. 12), yet how often do nurses describe older clients as demented? Ann responds to this, stating it is *horrendous ... implying something which is not human* (Sabat et al., 2011, p. 12). In fact, far from nursing older people being a low-skilled speciality, it requires exceptional interpersonal, assessment and care-giving skills, as providing high-quality elder care is about retaining the personhood of someone who may not be able to communicate verbally.

Terms used in healthcare, such as 'feeders', 'bed blockers', 'the old' and 'the stroke in bed 10' can also serve to dehumanise individuals, and may result in the depersonalisation of the individual who is referred to. The report *Seeing the Patient in the Person* (Kings Fund, 2008) challenges the NHS to see the person rather than the patient. This was further endorsed by the Francis review, which stressed *if there is one lesson to be learnt, I suggest it is that people must always come before numbers. It is the individual experience ... that really matters* (Francis, 2011, p. 4).

Implications for nursing care

In order to explore the implications of dehumanisation upon nursing care, let us reconsider Molly and Frank's latest experience.

Case study of Molly and Frank, part 3

Molly felt very unwell in hospital and spent most of her time lying in bed. Frank visited every day without fail (during the visiting hours of 2–8 p.m.). He would either drive himself or occasionally his best friend would bring him in to see Molly. Frank often noticed that her food was left at her side, relatively untouched and out of her reach. One day when Frank went in, he noticed the soup in the plastic beaker was cold and Molly had again hardly touched her dinner. Frank was becoming increasingly worried about Molly, who was not her normal self, so he went to talk to a member of staff. Frank admitted to not really understanding who wore which uniform but found a young woman with a red tabard and asked her about Molly. She replied, 'I can't help you – I don't know who she is', and walked away.

Whether the woman in the red tabard was a nurse, a healthcare assistant or a domestic, she should have taken Frank to the right person for help. Anyone working in a supermarket will stop what they are doing and direct customers to what they seek. As consumers we expect certain standards of customer service: should this not be equally as important or even more so in healthcare? Patients and their families are people, not tasks. Molly may have been seen as a 'patient' and a 'task to be done' rather than as a person.

Nay (2010) writes about nursing as an 'I–thou' or 'I–it' occupation; in 'I–thou', it is a relationship between two people and as such the person is recognised and valued as an individual. In contrast, the 'I–it' occupation focuses on a body and a task to be done. Whilst this case study raises many issues regarding communication within the nursing team, it may also have been that Molly was seen as a 'feeder' as she required assistance, thus denoting her to an 'I–it' status and simply another task to be undertaken in addition to an already long list. Assigning Molly as a task and not a person may mean that she is not prioritised, resulting in many days her food being left untouched or out of her reach. In order to provide good-quality care to older people nurses must view nursing as an 'I–thou' occupation and focus upon the people they are working with, as opposed to seeing tasks to be done. Ultimately, providing good-quality care is about focusing on patients as individuals, rather than dehumanising them and seeing them as a task to be done.

Stereotyping

Judging people on the basis of the assumptions held about them is called stereotyping; these judgements are often based upon the belief that all members within that group are the same. For instance, there is a stereotype that nurses are women and doctors are men, and that male nurses are gay, although this is far from the truth. Stereotyping leads to unfair and detrimental generalisations about individuals. The difficulty with stereotypes is that individuals are often unaware that they hold these beliefs unless they are challenged.

Activity 3.3 — *Reflection*

Take a moment and consider yourself in the future, when you are 75 years old. Either draw a picture or write a list of words which you feel will describe you then.

As this is a personal reflection, no outline answer is supplied.

Student nurses undertaking this activity frequently include a walking stick, walking frame or a coffin or gravestone; there are very few drawings of themselves as active or independent. This is because the stereotype of older people is someone who is frail, senile, confused, incontinent, cantankerous, feeble and boring. We are exposed to these stereotypes of older people through things like traffic signs which depict a hunched-up figure leaning heavily on a walking stick, through the media which often reflect a frail, confused or cantankerous figure as well as through humour – think how few birthday cards depict a positive image of ageing.

Implications for nursing care

One of the major implications of stereotyping is the notion of self-fulfilling prophecy: if older people are expected to behave in certain ways, and are perceived with certain attributes then they quickly only behave in those ways with those attributes. This can be explained by examining the work *The Unpopular Patient* by Stockwell (1972).

Research summary: *The Unpopular Patient* by Stockwell (1972)

This research was one of a group of research projects funded by the Department of Health and sponsored by the Royal College of Nursing. The study was exploring interpersonal relationships between nurses and patients in general wards. The study identified that patients on a ward were either 'popular' or 'unpopular' with the nurses. Patients were assessed as either 'good' or 'bad' depending upon how 'demanding', 'attention seeking' or 'cooperative' they were deemed to be, and this affected the way that nurses interacted, or otherwise, with them.

The study found that 'good' patients were rewarded with the nurses' attention and time; they were more 'liked' by the nursing team and positive words were used to describe them. In contrast, 'unpopular' patients were labelled as 'uncooperative' and 'demanding' and were effectively 'punished' by the negative words that were used to describe them, as well as by a lack of attention by the nurses who even sometimes ignored them or disconnected their call bell.

As nurses we need to consider and maybe challenge some of the stereotypes we hold of older people. If nurses hold stereotypes of older people as difficult, confused or cantankerous before they have even entered a relationship with them, then they already have a negative label. Conversely, if older people are considered passive, then having an older person who is assertive in interactions with staff may also be perceived negatively.

Welfarism and medicalisation

One of the largest stereotypes healthcare practitioners have of older people is that they are frail and require health and/or social care services. This is called welfarism – a tendency to assume that individuals require welfare services on the basis of belonging to a certain group. Nurses can get a very distorted and negative perspective of ageing, for while the majority of older people nurses see in healthcare are ill or require support, there is a greater number of older people who nurses do not see, as they are living active, independent lives. The problem associated with welfarism is that it can lead to practitioners taking a paternalistic role with clients, disempowering them by assuming that they have to make decisions for older people who are unable to make these for themselves.

The process of medicalisation works in a similar way. In this context it usually refers to the attribution of a medical diagnosis to a particular state, such as distress, so instead of recognising that somebody is upset and providing comfort, professionals may label them as 'depressed' and prescribe drugs. Nationally there has been a move towards standardising care using care pathways (such as the Liverpool care pathways, falls care pathways, fractured neck of femur care pathways) in order to provide high-quality, cost-effective care. But these approaches focus upon a medical disease and can lose sight of the person concerned. How often in healthcare do we refer to people as their medical diagnosis ('diabetic patient', 'stroke victim', 'deliberate self-harmer')? These are examples of medicalisation, and result in nurses focusing upon the disease rather than the individual living with it. Instead of referring to a diabetic patient, nurses need to refer to a person living with diabetes; these very simple adjustments reframe our mind to see the person and not the diagnosis first.

Implications for nursing care

If we assume that older people are frail and require support, we may not seek their opinions regarding their care or help them make an informed choice. It is vital when nursing older people that we respect their autonomy, as enshrined in the Nursing and Midwifery Council Code (2008). They have the right to make choices about their care, and for their choices to be respected so long as they have capacity. If nurses fail to respect older people's autonomy and facilitate their choice, then learned helplessness can occur.

The process of learned helplessness can develop from any experience a person perceives as difficult, challenging or negative (Seligman, 1975, cited by Rungapadiachy, 1999). It occurs in situations where people feel they have no control; this makes people feel helpless as they believe they cannot do anything to change the situation. This is both physically and psychologically draining and reduces motivation. From this experience comes a general belief that they would not be able to change similar situations in the future, irrespective of whether they could or not. They therefore learn to become helpless: see the case study of Lily, below.

Case study of Lily

Imagine your elderly aunt Lily, who has recently moved into a care home as she requires ongoing support, due to her confusion resulting from her dementia. At home Lily used to have a snack about 9.30, as she is an early riser. Lily is sat in the day room in the home, and the carers are busy assisting other residents. Lily tells one of the carers that she is hungry and asks them to get her a snack. The carer responds, 'Hold on a moment, Lily, I will be back to see you in five minutes'. However the carer does not come back. Lily tries another member of staff who also responds in a similar fashion. After three attempts Lily gives up and just sits quietly in the day room. The next morning the carers are assisting Lily to get dressed and Lily informs them she would like to wear her pink dress, to which the nurse replies, 'Oh Lily, it's cold out today, trousers would be best'.

From looking at Lily's experience it is clear to see how these two separate incidents could make Lily feel that she doesn't have a voice regarding her own care, and therefore she may simply give up and become passive, letting the nurses and carers make decisions for her, and in doing so learns to become helpless.

Infantilisation and elderspeak

Infantilisation occurs when there is a mismatch between an individual's ability to communicate and others' perception of that ability (Brown and Draper, 2003). In the case of older people, this is reinforced by negative perceptions and stereotypes in which ageing is associated with mental decline, resulting in practitioners using patronising and inappropriate terms of address. Salari (2005) identified four different types of infantilisation: speech, behaviour, activity and environmental.

Speech infantilisation

Speech infantilisation, sometimes referred to as elderspeak (Williams et al., 2004), is the process by which clients are given the status of children through the language used by some practitioners, based on the stereotype of older people being less competent than younger people (Williams et al., 2004). Speech infantilisation can be very disempowering for older people and occurs in at least five ways:

1. using overly familiar terms without the person's consent, such as 'sweetie', 'love', 'dear', 'darling';
2. through the use of simple and/or childish vocabulary and simplified grammar: 'Mary, you are on the bed pan, do a wee wee for me please';
3. the use of collective pronouns, such as 'Let's have a bath, shall we?';
4. calling someone by their first name without their permission;
5. talking over a client or referring to them in the third person.

Let us consider this further by reading Susan's experience.

Case study of Susan

Susan was admitted to the ward to investigate her abdominal pain. She is registered blind, having lost her sight in her early childhood, and walks with a white stick. Also present was Susan's daughter, Tina. During the admission to the ward the nurses posed all of their questions to Tina and ignored Susan. They asked Tina, 'How does she manage with her shopping?', at which point Susan responded, 'She *manages fine, thank you!'*

In this example you can see how the nurses have infantilised Susan by talking over her even though she was perfectly capable of answering their questions.

Speech infantilisation is often made worse by the way people talk, such as in a high pitch, with exaggerated intonation and pronunciation, as well as loud, slow speech. Good communication demands you speak clearly with all patients, especially the elderly, but not in a patronising way.

Behaviour infantilisation

This refers to the public disclosure of conditions, such as whether someone has had their bowels open, which for older people can be compounded by speech infantilisation. It also refers to enforced wake and sleep times; this can occur in both acute and residential settings, telling older people, 'It's time for bed now' rather than asking them, as adults, what time they would like to go to bed. Behaviour infantilisation also includes reprimands and/or punishments as an incentive for good behaviour, for example, 'Let's have a bath and then I'll make you a nice cup of tea'. Note here the lack of choice, especially as the speech is often accompanied by a guiding arm under the elbow. Lastly, not listening is another example of behaviour infantilisation, so instead of the nurse really listening to what the person is saying, just nodding and responding mechanistically, 'I know, it's terrible isn't it?'

Activity infantilisation

Activity infantilisation refers to involving older people in child-oriented activities, such as playing with toys, colouring with crayons, listening to children's music or watching children's television programmes. Also included within this could be a focus upon childhood memories rather than adult accomplishments. Choice is a central component of activity infantilisation in that older people feel they have no choice but to participate.

Environment infantilisation

This refers to any child-oriented decor such as Easter-themed decorations, in which there are large Easter bunnies delivering Easter eggs in a residential or day care setting. Lack of privacy is also part of environment infantilisation and this is especially pertinent within a hospital setting, as often hospital staff do not perceive the curtains as a barrier and will open them and walk through without recognising or respecting the person's right to privacy behind them.

Implications for nursing care

Giles et al. (1993, cited by Brown and Draper, 2003) researched infantilisation among 60 older people, and their findings are shown in Table 3.1.

As we can see from Table 3.1, infantilisation is a major issue affecting older people, which may increase their experience of feeling vulnerable within a health or social care setting. Therefore,

- 57% believed that older adults in general were spoken to in this way
- 36% believed it happened often
- 59% claimed they had experienced such talk personally
- 13% claimed it happened often
- 58% felt patronised
- 50% felt irritated
- 17% felt angry
- 15% were made to feel inferior

Table 3.1: Research on infantilisation and older people

we need to examine critically the way we speak and act with older people to ensure we respect them as autonomous adults rather than treating them in a childlike way.

Safeguarding

Another way of seeing vulnerability of older people is within the context of abuse, that a person is in some way vulnerable to being abused.

No Secrets, the safeguarding policy related to vulnerable adults, was published by the Department of Health in 2000. It noted that health and social care staff have to work in partnership to ensure that policies and procedures are in place to protect vulnerable adults. Within this document abuse was identified as: *violation of an individual's human and civil rights by any other person or persons* (Department of Health, 2000).

Further clarification was provided, denoting that abuse can:

- be a single or repeated act;
- be intentional or unintentional;
- happen in any relationship;
- result in significant harm or exploitation.

However, many practitioners may struggle to define a human and civil right, so this may not be a useful definition. Any definition should be instantly understandable by staff. Here is the definition of Action on Elder Abuse, a national charity, which is clearer: *A single or repeated act or lack of appropriate action, occurring within any relationship where there is an expectation of trust, which causes harm or distress to an older person* (Action on Elder Abuse, 2003).

The *No Secrets* policy also defined a vulnerable adult as: *Anyone aged 18 years+ who is or may be in need of community care services by reason of mental or other disability, age or illness and who is or may be unable to take care of him/herself* (Department of Health, 2000, pp. 8–9).

Groups of people identified as vulnerable in the *No Secrets* document included older people, people with learning disabilities, people with physical disabilities, traumatic brain injuries or acquired brain damage and people with mental health problems. These guidelines have also been supported by the Safeguarding Vulnerable Groups Act 2006, which also recognised that people in residential accommodation or receiving domiciliary care, and people accessing healthcare or if they have difficulties managing their affairs because of a cognitive disorder are also vulnerable to abuse. There have been limited national studies into the abuse of older people. The Department of Health and Comic Relief commissioned one such piece of work, which identified that 2.6 per cent of the total UK population (aged over 66) reported experiencing maltreatment (O'Keeffe et al., 2007); however, this estimate must be received cautiously as many older people who experience abuse may not say, either because they decide not to, or because they are unable. The research also identified a correlation between increased incidence of abuse and poorer health status; thus people who were more dependent upon others were also more likely to be abused. Reasons for this may include increased dependency upon services, increased social isolation and maybe increased difficulties in communicating. The *No Secrets* policy was presented as an example of best practice, and is not enforceable by law, despite calls from charities such as Action on Elder Abuse, which argues that safeguarding vulnerable adults should have the same priority as safeguarding vulnerable children. Professionals and the public have also called for legalisation to protect vulnerable adults (Department of Health, 2009d).

The safeguarding agenda and disempowerment

However, there are problems associated with the term 'vulnerability' being aligned to safeguarding because this perspective of vulnerability is restrictive and potentially negative. This can lead to vulnerability being associated with terms such as weakness, failure, inequality, inferiority and dependence (Batchelor, 2006). In addition, Penhale and Parker (2008) argue that it also attaches a *victim status* to the individual which appears to apportion blame to them rather than the person, agency or society perpetuating the abuse. Due to these concerns the term 'protecting vulnerable adults' was superseded by 'safeguarding adults', to reflect that vulnerable adults are not different people – they are us, and all human beings can potentially be vulnerable (Eastman, 2008). The perception of the term 'vulnerable adult' as patronising and disempowering was further highlighted in the consultation of the *No Secrets* guidance (Department of Health, 2009d). In addition, this review also identified that the NHS was struggling with regard to safeguarding, seeing it as a social service responsibility. Coupled with a lack of adult safeguarding systems in the NHS, this has led to national guidance being developed for staff in the NHS (Department of Health, 2011a).

Implications for nursing practice

The Nursing and Midwifery Council Code of Conduct (2008) identifies that nurses have a professional responsibility to safeguard vulnerable adults. Their responsibility is to act without delay if they (or a colleague) are putting someone at risk or if the environment in which they work is putting people at risk. In line with their professional accountability, all nurses have a professional responsibility to follow their local trust adult safeguarding policy (Activity 3.4).

Activity 3.4 — ***Critical thinking***

Think back over your practice and identify individual clients who you felt may have been at risk of abuse. Next locate and read your local trust adult safeguarding policy and meet with the adult safeguarding lead for your trust. Discuss with them the local policy and procedure for raising concerns. Now think back to the person who you previously thought was at risk: should you have done anything differently? If so, write brief notes about what you would do now if you were presented with a similar situation again.

As this is a personal reflection, no outline answer is supplied.

Within this answer you should have identified that you must take action if you are concerned someone is at risk in line with your professional accountability, and spoken to your line manager or local safeguarding lead. There isn't the scope within this chapter to explore this in more detail. As such you need to access and read *Safeguarding Adults: The role of health service practitioners* (Department of Health, 2011a).

Mutual vulnerability

Nursing as a profession is not risk-free: it is physically, emotionally and spiritually demanding. Physically, nurses work long days in very stressful environments; the work is emotionally demanding as nurses work with people who are experiencing distress, and for whom a prognosis may not always be positive. This, coupled with the emotional labour that is involved with nursing in emotionally engaging with people who are vulnerable, can make it very tiring. In addition, seeing people in distress who are ill may lead nurses to face questions regarding their own morbidity and mortality. So it can be argued that nursing can itself make us feel vulnerable. At the start of the chapter, vulnerability was linked to harm and wounding, which can be physical or psychological. Many nurses experience this sense of wounding because of the emotional commitment that the role brings. Therefore we have a shared or mutual vulnerability with patients for whom we care.

Heaslip and Board (2012) undertook research with carers in a care home for people with dementia. They identified that many of the staff experienced feeling vulnerable for many reasons.

First, the staff were reminded of their own morbidity and mortality – indeed, within the home there was a resident who was only a couple of years older than some of the staff, and this was a stark reminder of their own human frailty.

It was evident that the staff really cared about the residents within the home and they had an emotional engagement with them. Dementia is a journey and at the end the person living with it enters the terminal phase; because of this journey the staff experienced multiple bereavements in grieving for the loss of the person they knew as the disease progressed, as well as the client's ultimate physical death.

People who have dementia can be unpredictable, depending on which area of the brain is affected. Some of the staff found it very difficult that during a single shift their relationship with the residents could change. For example, one of the healthcare assistants noted a resident she worked with well, and found that during a space of 30 minutes the carer went from being someone the resident liked and enjoyed being with to someone the resident was swearing at. The carer found this very distressing, as she did not know what she had done wrong.

The staff established a close relationship with the residents and their families; indeed, they saw themselves as part of that extended family, and they emotionally invested in the relationship and thus opened themselves up to wounding and feeling vulnerable.

The staff had a close relationship with residents and saw them very much as people; the nature of the care environment meant that they knew each person very well and this increased their emotional vulnerability.

Stenbock-Hult and Sarvimäki (2011) identified vulnerability as both a resource and a burden. As a burden, vulnerability is associated with the risk of being harmed (experiencing pain, feeling under pressure and feeling insecure) as well as protecting oneself either by hiding or dissociating from the job. Earlier in the chapter we explored dehumanisation, infantilisation, welfarism and stereotyping; staff may use these processes as ways of protecting themselves from feeling vulnerable, as it is easier to disengage from the emotional aspect of the role and focus upon the physical role or the task to be undertaken. Recent high-profile cases such as the Winterbourne View review (Flynn, 2012b) and Mid Staffordshire NHS Trust inquiry (Healthcare Commission, 2009; Francis, 2011), as well as numerous *Panorama* programmes, have highlighted examples of poor care. We must consider whether the nurses and care staff involved have simply 'switched off' their emotions and no longer see the person they are caring for; this may happen when it is simply too painful for them to care emotionally. In an effort to reduce our own vulnerability we must make sure we do not increase the vulnerability of the clients in our care.

In contrast, Stenbock-Hult and Sarvimäki (2011) also perceive vulnerability as a resource, and this includes recognising and acknowledging our own feelings and using them as a benchmark for actions, in order to enhance the care that clients receive.

Implications for nursing care

Nurses must be self-aware and have the courage to find a voice, to become the client's advocate and speak up for clients within the service. This speaking up can be at a personal level of challenging poor practice of their peers, at a cultural level of creating a culture where high-quality personalised care is valued or even at a structural level, challenging poor staffing levels which affect the quality of care (Figure 3.2).

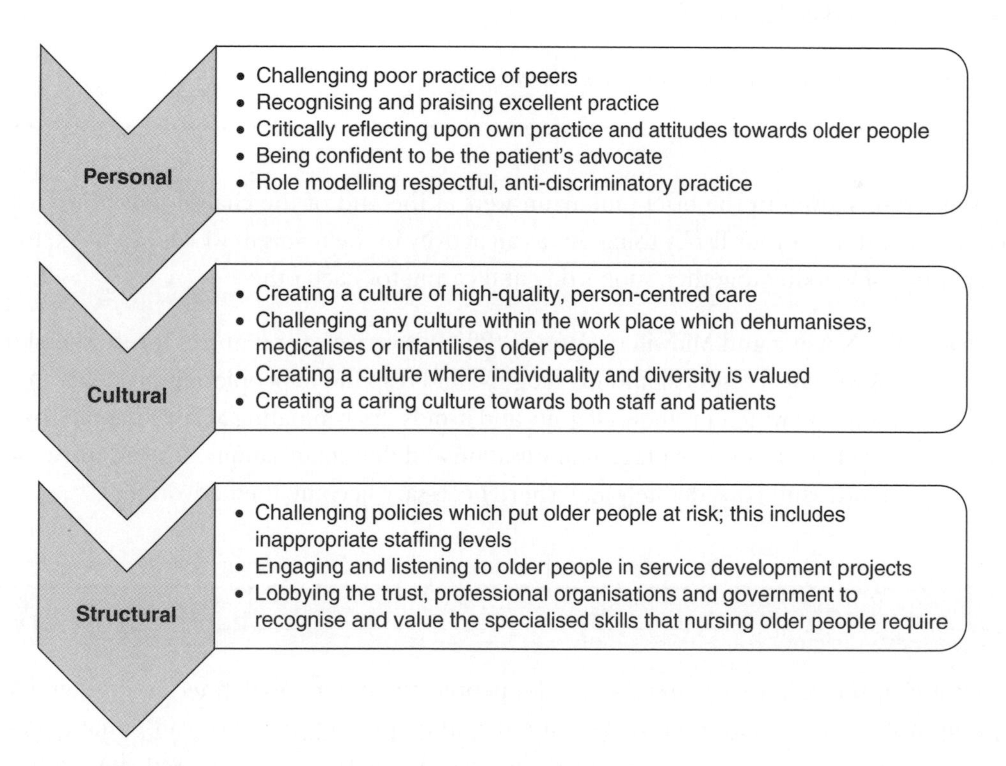

Figure 3.2: The ways nurses can promote high-quality care

The senses framework

Nolan (1997) (cited by Nolan et al., 2006a) identified the senses framework for both staff and clients; this can be used to identify ways to ensure that staff and patients feel supported and cared for, which will in turn assist them in managing feelings of vulnerability. The senses framework includes:

- sense of security – to feel safe and receive quality care;
- sense of continuity – recognition of one's past to make sense of the present and to plan for the future;
- sense of belonging – opportunities to form relationships and feel part of the community;
- sense of purpose – opportunities to engage in purposeful activity, goals to aim for;
- sense of fulfilment – to achieve valued goals and to feel satisfied with one's efforts;
- sense of significance – to feel that you, and what you do, matter. You feel valued as a person of worth.

Activity 3.5 *Critical thinking*

Study the senses framework. Make a list of activities you could undertake to enhance these senses:

- for patients and their families;
- for staff and colleagues.

An outline answer is provided at the end of the chapter.

The suggestions given in the brief outline answers at the end of the chapter are by no means exclusive. Build upon your list by using this as an activity in the teams in which you work, to create a culture of working together, supporting and caring for each other.

Ultimately, the Nursing and Midwifery Council (2008) is very clear on nurses' professional obligations, in that we have a responsibility to recognise and respond to people as individuals, providing personalised care which promotes dignity and avoids discriminating against people (by processes such as welfarism, stereotyping, infantilisation and dehumanisation). Instead nurses must treat people kindly and considerately and where necessary become their advocate.

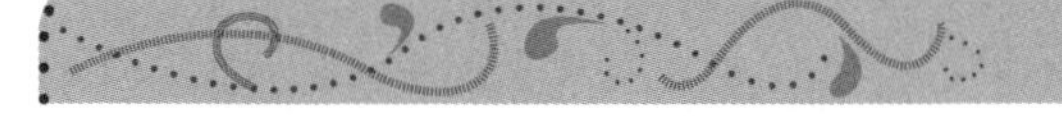

Chapter summary

In this chapter we have examined why older people are sometimes defined as a vulnerable group within society. However we have also begun to question this and realise that not all older people may experience feeling vulnerable. We have also recognised that feeling vulnerable can either be created or compounded by the interaction between care staff and older people themselves and begun to explore how some processes of discrimination may induce feelings of vulnerability, namely dehumanisation, welfarism, stereotyping and infantilisation.

We continued to examine how some older people may be more vulnerable to abuse and examined the national guidance with regard to safeguarding. Through the activities readers will be better informed regarding their local process and lead for safeguarding in their trust or department.

Lastly, we examined how the staff themselves may experience vulnerability and how, in an attempt to reduce their own feelings of vulnerability, staff may inadvertently increase the experience of vulnerability of others. The activity in this section was geared towards enabling readers to develop strategies within their organisation to support not only older people and their families but also themselves and their colleagues, so vulnerability is seen as a resource instead of perceived as a burden.

Activities: brief outline answers

Activity 3.1

Groups commonly identified as vulnerable are:

- older people;
- children;
- people with mental health issues;
- people with a physical or learning disability;
- people from ethnic minorities;
- people who are homeless.

These groups of people may have been identified as vulnerable because:

- they are reliant upon other people;
- they have poor physical health;
- they have poor mental health;
- they experience difficulty communicating their needs;
- they may be socially isolated;
- they are financially insecure.

Activity 3.2

Crabbit Old Woman	
Etic	**Emic**
Lines 3, 4–5, 9–10	Lines 18–33, 35–38

Activity 3.5

Senses	Patients and their families	Staff and colleagues
Sense of security – to feel safe and receive quality care	Listen to patient and/or family's concerns Show family where their loved ones are when asked, or find someone to answer their questions Respect patients' dignity Treat people how we would wish to be treated	Work as a team, supporting each other Create a culture in the work place in which each member of staff is valued Share your knowledge with your peers and be receptive to learning theirs Treat each other with respect
Sense of continuity – recognition of one's past to make sense of the present and to plan for the future	Support them in recognising that this current illness may not go on forever Question how they have managed previous life transitions, focusing upon the skills they already have Support them in making plans for the future Involve older people and their families in discharge planning	Enable a culture where people can express their feelings, their sadness and frustration When clients die, enable staff to talk about what happened and support them whilst they make sense of their feelings Have a vision for the service in which all staff contribute
Sense of belonging – opportunities to form relationships and feel part of the community	Ensure the patients and their families know the layout of the ward, for example where the kitchen is, and that it is OK to make themselves a drink Provide information regarding the routines of the care environment Invest in the therapeutic relationship; be interested in patients and their families as individuals Offer opportunities to talk to other people in the care environment	Treat your colleagues with respect Value each team member's contribution and commend each other on jobs done well Maybe have social events where the team can come together and get to know each other Celebrate special events in each other's lives
Sense of purpose – opportunities to engage in purposeful activity, goals to aim for	Support people in making sense of what is happening to them Dependent upon the environment, enable individuals to participate in activities which give meaning to their lives Ask patients and their families what their goals are and build this into care-planning arrangements	Enable staff to feel they have a voice where they can make suggestions to enhance the care or working environment Enable opportunities for staff development and/or training
Sense of fulfilment – to achieve valued goals and to feel satisfied with one's efforts	To revisit goals and identify where achievements have been made and celebrate these Remember we do not 'do to', rather we 'work with'	Identify occurrences when the team have made positive contributions to individuals' lives Celebrate work done well

Senses	Patients and their families	Staff and colleagues
Sense of significance – to feel that you, and what you do, matter. You feel valued as a person of worth	Remember to see the person, and not the patient. Every person we care for is loved and treasured by someone and we must remember this. Value and respect our fellow human beings	Remember to see each other as individuals as well as team members Focus upon people's strengths and positive contributions whilst supporting them to continue to develop Celebrate each other's special times

Useful websites

The following websites offer a wealth of further reading and information regarding safeguarding older people from abuse.

Action on Elder Abuse: http://www.elderabuse.org.uk

Department of Health Safeguarding Adults, the role of Health Services: http://www.dh.gov.uk/en/Publicationsandstatistics/Publications/PublicationsPolicyAndGuidance/DH_124882

Nursing and Midwifery Council: http://www.nmc-uk.org/Nurses-and-midwives

Office of Public Sector Information. Safeguarding Vulnerable Groups Act. Available from http://www.opsi.gov.uk/acts/acts/2006/en/06en47-c.htm

Social Care Institute for Excellence: http://www.scie.org.uk/adults/safeguarding/index.asp

Further reading

Heaslip, V, and Ryden, J (2013) *Understanding Vulnerability: A nursing and healthcare approach.* Oxford: Wiley Blackwell.

Mandelstram, M (2009) *Safeguarding Vulnerable Adults and the Law.* London: Jessica Kingsley Publishers (to read more about safeguarding).

Thompson, N (2003) *Promoting Equality.* Basingstoke: Palgrave Macmillan (to read more about the processes of discrimination).

Chapter 4
Nursing for well-being in later life

Ann Hemingway and Rosalind Green

NMC Standards for Pre-registration Nursing Education

Domain 1: Professional values

2. All nurses must practise in a holistic, non-judgmental, caring and sensitive manner that avoids assumptions, supports social inclusion; recognises and respects individual choice; and acknowledges diversity. Where necessary, they must challenge inequality, discrimination and exclusion from access to care.
3. All nurses must support and promote the health, wellbeing, rights and dignity of people, groups, communities and populations. These include people whose lives are affected by ill health, disability, ageing, death and dying. Nurses must understand how these activities influence public health.
4. All nurses must work in partnership with service users, carers, families, groups, communities and organisations. They must manage risk, and promote health and well-being while aiming to empower choices that promote self-care and safety.

Domain 2: Communication and interpersonal skills

1. All nurses must build partnerships and therapeutic relationships through safe, effective and non-discriminatory communication. They must take account of individual differences, capabilities and needs.
2. All nurses must use a range of communication skills and technologies to support person-centred care and enhance quality and safety. They must ensure people receive all the information they need in a language and manner that allows them to make informed choices and share decision making. They must recognise when language interpretation or other communication support is needed and know how to obtain it.
4. All nurses must recognise when people are anxious or in distress and respond effectively, using therapeutic principles, to promote their wellbeing, manage personal safety and resolve conflict. They must use effective communication strategies and negotiation techniques to achieve best outcomes, respecting the dignity and human rights of all concerned. They must know when to consult a third party and how to make referrals for advocacy, mediation or arbitration.
5. All nurses must use therapeutic principles to engage, maintain and, where appropriate, disengage from professional caring relationships, and must always respect professional boundaries.

6. All nurses must take every opportunity to encourage health-promoting behaviour through education, role modelling and effective communication.

Domain 3: Nursing practice and decision making

8. All nurses must provide educational support, facilitation skills and therapeutic nursing interventions to optimise health and wellbeing. They must promote self-care and management whenever possible, helping people to make choices about their healthcare needs, involving families and carers where appropriate, to maximise their ability to care for themselves.

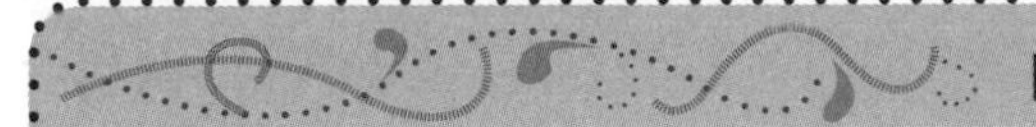

NMC Essential Skills Clusters (ESCs)

This chapter will support the following ESCs:

Cluster: Care, compassion and communication

2. People can trust the newly registered graduate nurse to engage in person centred care empowering people to make choices about how their needs are met when they are unable to meet them themselves.
3. People can trust the newly registered graduate nurse to respect them as individuals and strive to help them preserve their dignity at all times.
5. People can trust the newly registered graduate nurse to engage with them in a warm, sensitive and compassionate way.

Chapter aims

By the end of this chapter you will be able to:

- understand the meaning of well-being and start to consider what that means in the context of caring and your responsibilities as a nurse;
- understand the humanisation framework (see Chapter 1) and how it can be used in practice to promote well-being and ensure safe and dignified care.

Introduction

This chapter will focus on defining well-being and its relevance for nursing older people. It will consider the findings from a discussion with retired nurses living in a care home environment, which focused on how to provide nursing care to promote well-being. The chapter will then discuss the suggested *humanising value framework* for nursing practice, created by Todres et al. (2009), and its relevance for the promotion of well-being in older people. We will look at the 'dimensions' proposed in this framework one by one, and collectively, as together they form a value base for considering the potentially humanising and dehumanising elements in nursing interactions. They will also be used to give examples of how nurses can promote well-being in older people in hospital.

Defining and promoting well-being in the caring environment

Activity 4.1 *Reflection*

Take a few minutes to think about how you would define 'wellbeing'. If you were the patient, and being nursed, would there be any elements of your definition which would be particularly important to you?

As this is a personal reflection, no outline answer is supplied.

Studies on well-being in the caring environment tend to agree on the main aspects of well-being, and this section of the chapter will be structured under these headings.

Autonomy and self-care

Mental and physical activity increase well-being and positive ageing, according to O'Sullivan and Hocking (2006); experiencing autonomy and being involved in self-care are important contributors to well-being. It is important that elderly patients are given the opportunity to help organise and undertake their own care, for example with cleaning, washing, getting dressed or being involved with organising activities or schedules, as this can lead to increased mental and physical activity. Gleibs et al. (2011) state that clubs may be a useful means of getting elderly people involved and engaged in meaningful ways, and these are necessary factors for well-being. They invited residents to join a gentlemen's or ladies' club and well-being improved for both men and women through attendance at the clubs.

Scenario

Imagine you are working in a care home where there are few opportunities for residents to develop autonomy and self-care. You want to start to develop such opportunities, and begin by talking to the other staff about how they would like to be involved. Two of the care staff, Jawinda and Cynthia, who have worked in the home for many years, tell you that there used to be meetings to discuss ways that residents could be actively involved, and they are keen to start these again as they knew it really helped the residents.

Occupation

We all know that older people like to be occupied: O'Sullivan and Hocking (2006) in their New Zealand study emphasise the impact of occupation in later life. They state that it is crucial that older people have the opportunity to engage in occupational activity to improve well-being, saying that *being occupied gives meaning to life and helps to create occupational routines that provide people with security [by giving] a natural subconscious rhythm to their day* (p. 350).

Relationships with carers, caring and well-being

As nurses, we need to make sure that the routine meeting of basic needs is carried out with a focus on dignity and respect, whether it is being done by nurses or healthcare assistants or other care staff under our supervision. We need to take notice of the way a person is handled, spoken to or ignored. Rees suggests that *the degree of sensitivity with which this care is delivered makes all the difference to a life fraught with degradation and discomfort and a poor sense of wellbeing, the manner in which these tasks are done is the most important thing in the world* (Rees, 2007, p. 45). The 'I am giving you food therefore you are being cared for' approach is not enough to create a sense of well-being. Caring is so much more than practical handling and must include the carer thinking about the person being cared for with an attitude of respect and kindness. Put yourself in the patient's place, or imagine this is your elderly father or mother. We know that shortage of time and heavy workload can impact negatively on attitudes to care, but as qualified professionals we need to combat this at all times. Rees argues that training should emphasise kindness and seeing the elderly person as a valued human being. The findings from the first and second Francis Reports (2009, 2013) have shown us that neglecting an emphasis on kindness and caring in nursing can result in greatly increased suffering for those we care for and their loved ones.

As nurses we always need to think about carers' experiences in the care home or hospital setting. Research reveals a complex interdependence of relationships between carers and clients, and the ethics of the carers and the organisation. Fagerberg and Engstrom's (2012) study, 'Care of the old: a matter of ethics, organization and relationships', concludes that lack of time is a factor in being involved and engaged with a client so that 'positive care' which promotes well-being takes place.

When residents are assessed to help understand their care needs, how to promote their well-being needs to be considered and planned for as part of their care. Research by Worden et al. (2005) revealed that 35 per cent of care homes studied did not assess for the social needs of residents. This is a concern since the social needs of residents are important for improving well-being and decreasing depression. More specifically, the data revealed that care homes are not addressing the domains in relation to the residents' own perspective; the domain of 'problems and issues in the user's own words' was not filled out in all 126 forms examined.

These studies so far have looked at different features of care and well-being promotion in the caring environment and their findings have highlighted the following areas as important for promoting well-being in this environment: autonomy and self-care, occupation and relationships with carers. We will now turn to a discussion with retired nurses on what well-being means for them when being cared for, and how to promote it.

What do retired nurses think of their nursing care?

All the retired nurses engaged in this (2012) discussion group were female and aged over 60, living in a nursing home environment. There were two questions for the group: firstly to explore the term well-being and what it means, and secondly, what the retired nurses felt they needed as recipients of care to enhance their well-being.

Overall what emerged from this discussion falls within three main themes (Table 4.1), through which well-being is defined and promoted through nursing care.

Comfort, security and freedom = well-being in the care home environment		
The key constituents of which are:		
Healthy relationships = Respect, safety, kindness, empathy, acceptance and negotiation	Freedom to choose = Food, activities, autonomy of movement	Creativity = Independence, social and physical outlets, achievement

Table 4.1: How retired nurses view well-being

Healthy relationships

It would appear that well-being can be promoted through meaningful contact with others. What form does respect take? How do we as human beings express it? This discussion suggests that respect is demonstrated when the other person's opinions and presence are acted upon with kindness and empathy, which in turn impacts positively on well-being. Participants who themselves had great experience as carers felt that respectful relations are likely to begin with the manager, and then through staff training and development and role modelling, this behaviour would be offered to those being cared for.

Another area of concern was safety. A sense of safety came from being confident that staff and others would be treating and speaking to residents in a kindly manner and with awareness of them as individuals. Interestingly, when staff were disrespectful, or ignored the presence or views of those they cared for, this made residents feel unsafe and vulnerable. Feelings of safety, security and comfort were engendered through being able to know and predict another person's behaviour towards them. This highlights the need for care to focus on not just physical comfort but also the experiences of clients in order to enable them to feel comfortable and at ease within their immediate environment and promote feelings of well-being.

The retired nurses saw empathy as an ability to put oneself in another person's shoes, which would in turn provide an understanding of why people behave as they do. Healthy meaningful relationships require empathy so that we can perceive needs in others and in particular why they want to behave in a certain way or do a certain activity. The subthemes of respect, empathy, acceptance, negotiation and safety as components of well-being found here all support Rees's (2007) and Fagerberg and Enstrom's (2012) findings. This also raises the question of how time is spent by staff? They need the skills to be able to spend time with those they care for in a respectful way whilst also seeing to the practical aspects of care (Rees, 2007).

Activity 4.2 | ***Critical thinking***

Take a few minutes to consider the issues of respect, empathy, acceptance, negotiation and safety. In the way you care for someone, how as a nurse can you practically demonstrate these qualities?

An outline answer is provided at the end of the chapter.

The discussion with the retired nurses found that an underlying value of acceptance was an important theme in well-being. An atmosphere of accepting everyone's varying needs and wishes should infuse any caring environment. Again, it was suggested that this could be achieved through shared activities and that those activities were important for being able to gain access to others and create meaning by meeting others and exchanging information through the web of relationships between carers and others.

Freedom to choose

This was discussed in a variety of ways and in various different situations, but was deemed very important to well-being. Rees (2007) points out that not only should maintenance of autonomy be encouraged within the caring arena, but also it acts as a crucial component in well-being. The freedom to say what I am going to do; what I am going to eat for dinner; and when I am going to rest or bathe is crucial. Choice equals autonomy and this can be achieved by allowing small decisions to take place within the caring environment. Removing choice on any level is equal to removing well-being (O'Sullivan and Hocking, 2006). This was of great concern to the retired nurses as they felt not only deprived of choice but through that they were also deprived of the chance to maintain their interests, independence, creative and social activities, which were a high priority for them.

Creativity

Chances of involvement in enriching activities were given a high significance by this group. O'Sullivan and Hocking (2006) cite the importance of being able to engage in an activity which provides meaning and is beneficial and instrumental in enhancing well-being. We discovered that the nature and quality of those chances for creative outlets were indeed a high priority in relation to maintaining and enhancing a sense of self-worth and well-being. A sense of achievement was furthered by creative outlets which were seen as a means of socialising and self-development, independence and pride.

Case study

Until recently Jo Norris was often visited by her close friend (and fellow rambler) Ann. However Ann is ill and suffering from Parkinson's disease which stops her coming to visit Jo in her flat as she can no longer drive and her ability to walk any distance is impaired.

Jo is a mother of three who has spent many years at home caring for her family. Jo's partner passed away ten years ago. In her 50s, Jo began to volunteer and work in a local charity shop. Jo has been a keen walker and rambler all her life and until recently had many friends through this activity and the local ramblers' association.

Jo also has kept an allotment for most of her adult life, which one of her daughters, who lives locally, has now taken on. Jo is now 75 and over the last few years has developed glaucoma in one eye and has a cataract in the other. This has limited Jo's confidence when walking outside and has meant that she can no longer volunteer in the local charity shop and no longer tend to her beloved allotment.

Two of Jo's children live in the UK with one, her son, living in Australia. Jo sees her family at Christmas and on her birthday; however she described her relationship with them as distant. Jo's partner was violent towards her and the children and as the children grew up they felt she should leave him and they had many disagreements about this over the years. Jo feels this has affected their relationships long-term and that it has stopped them from being closer as a family.

Jo can no longer afford to run a car and is living on a state pension. She owns a flat (two-bedroom, second floor) but has very little disposable income and no savings and feels that this stops her from getting out. On top of which, with her failing sight she has lost her confidence about using public transport.

You meet Jo when she is admitted to hospital for eye surgery for glaucoma.

The humanising framework

We will now consider the different dimensions of what it means to be human within a caring context, using the humanising framework proposed by Todres et al. (2009) (Table 4.2).

Forms of humanisation	Forms of dehumanisation
Insiderness	Objectification
Agency	Passivity
Uniqueness	Homogenisation
Togetherness	Isolation
Sense making	Loss of meaning
Personal journey	Loss of personal journey
Sense of place	Dislocation
Embodiment	Reductionist body

Table 4.2: The dimensions of humanisation/dehumanisation (Todres et al., 2009)

How can we ensure we are offering humanised care to Jo, in such a way that we actively promote her well-being? We will discuss the framework, and how it affects nursing Jo, under each of the 'dimensions' proposed in the framework.

Insiderness versus objectification

To be human is to experience life in relation to how you are; your feelings, mood and emotions are all a lens through which you experience the world. We need to focus not on patient problems but their abilities (skills, knowledge, motivation) and potential so that we do not treat people like objects, problems, needs or diseases.

Activity 4.3 *Reflection*

Take a few minutes to think about how often we as nurses see a patient with dementia as a list of fragmented risks and issues rather than as an individual who has the potential to be actively involved in solving problems. This problem-based disempowering focus does not lead to a positive shared vision of care but a dependency upon the nurse to make decisions. Have you ever viewed patients in this way, or observed other nurses doing so? What can you do to avoid this?

As this is a personal reflection, no outline answer is supplied.

Agency versus passivity

As humans we make choices and are generally held accountable for our actions. We do not commonly see ourselves as totally passive or totally determined but instead have the potential to live and act within limits; seeing ourselves as having a sense of choice or freedom appears to be linked to our social, physical and mental health (Stansfeld et al., 2002). Patients can be seen as passive recipients of nursing care or as problems waiting to be solved or treated and this may result in them becoming disempowered. Ensuring we maintain our patients' sense of control offers another way of viewing individuals; this then helps us to make sure that choice and accountability are woven into our interactions and interventions. We have to consider what possibilities exist to enable individuals to take matters into their own hands and self-manage their care.

Activity 4.4 *Decision making*

If you can offer Jo choice and a sense of agency (a sense that she has the ability to influence what is happening to her), then you are actively promoting her well-being. In relation to caring for Jo on the eye surgery unit, how can you ensure you are enabling choice and a sense of control wherever possible? What practical actions can you take?

An outline answer is provided at the end of the chapter.

Uniqueness versus homogenisation

Our uniqueness as human beings can never be reduced to a list of general characteristics such as age, gender and ethnicity. Each of us is unique, in relation to our relationships and our context, and this is how we see ourselves. An excessive focus on how our uniqueness is de-emphasised to enable us to fit into a group, such as diabetic, smokers, obese, socially isolated, can encourage a 'one size fits all' approach to care which separates individuals from the context of their life. When we need to focus on patients' problems in order to treat them, we should always consider the individual context, the patient's carers, friends, family and home, to counterbalance any generalisations we make which hide the characteristics that make individuals who they are. The complexities of their individual life may affect their ability to change their health, or self-care behaviour, and this is vital for us to consider if we are to be effective in our care.

Case study

Sharon is nursing Jo on the eye surgery unit. Sharon treats Jo as a unique human being who lives within a specific context which she knows best. Thinking of practical actions she can take to ensure this, Sharon shows Jo she is interested in her as a unique individual, and this will actively promoting her well-being.

Sharon listens to Jo and finds out about what she can and cannot do and what her wishes are in relation to her care. In addition she finds out about Jo's home circumstances and her life in order to help to plan her discharge safely. Sharon discusses what Jo will and will not be able to do following surgery and on discharge and what help she may need.

Togetherness versus isolation

To be human is to be unique individuals who are part of a community. Social isolation can have a negative impact on our health, although negative relationships may also cause us harm. Research indicates that social isolation impacts negatively on outcomes of chronic physical and psychological disease (Drennan et al., 2008). As nurses working within care settings we need to be acutely aware of the importance of social interaction between nurses and patients, as well as between patients and their carers, friends or family. In addition, we need to develop and maintain trust between all care staff and patients, which is paramount, and a central aspect of that is the maintenance of the individual's dignity.

Activity 4.5 — *Critical thinking*

If you were caring for Jo on the eye surgery unit, how could you ensure you are considering her social contacts outside the hospital so that she feels supported on the unit? Providing Jo with social contact and building a relationship with her during her stay will actively support her well-being. What practical actions can you take to ensure this?

There is an outline answer at the end of the chapter.

Sense making versus loss of meaning

To be human is to care about the meaning of our individual experiences. It matters far more to us that we are unhappy about our weight than understanding which percentile of the population for body mass index we fall into statistically (Hemingway, 2012). The immediacy of the search for meaning for many outweighs the significance of the search for statistical truth. When we are organising care we can categorise the experiences of individuals (ward from outpatients, day surgery to caring for people at home), but this ignores the holistic needs of people. There is no 'average person', so when we are treated as a number or statistic, our treatment or prevention opportunities may not make sense; what is significant statistically does not necessarily make sense to our human experience. Individuals may make sense of their health and well-being by looking at where and how they live rather than through official presentations of health risks and problems. As nurses we need to help people understand the issues in a way that empowers them and builds on their existing strengths.

Personal journey versus loss of personal journey

Human beings move through time in a meaningful way; we position ourselves in terms of our past, our present and our future. We are familiar with our past and could be ambivalent, fearful, excited or bored by our future. The experiences of health and healthcare that someone has are only a part of that person's life, but we need to recognise the distress caused by the interruption or threat caused by illness. If we always label our patients negatively, as needy or problematic, we do nothing for their sense of pride and engagement with past, present and future. Indeed, this approach could be seen as both disempowering and disabling.

Sense of place versus dislocation

To be human is to come from a particular place; our home is not just a collection of objects or experiences, it offers us security, comfort and familiarity. In addition spaces can provide a flourishing environment for bonds and connections between people (Hemingway and Stevens, 2011); an example is a day room, social area or garden where patients can engage with each other or with nature. Well-being cannot be separated from the place, the atmosphere and rhythms created by the built and natural environment, in all its varied manifestations. Too little attention has been paid to the quality of space within our homes and communities for eating and exercising, which contributes to unhealthily lifestyles impacting upon our physical health as a nation (Hemingway, 2012). The independent effect of place and residence on health cannot be ignored; arguably the only way to intervene successfully is to be ready to listen to what makes up a sense of home and place for individuals. Indeed, some researchers (Martinsen, 2006) have said that space and architecture are preservers of human dignity, particularly in care settings.

Activity 4.6 — *Critical thinking*

Read Jo's case study again, and suggest ways that as her nurse you can ensure that your care maintains Jo's dignity.

An outline answer is given at the end of the chapter.

Embodiment versus reductionist view of the body

We experience the world through our body in a positive or negative way. An assumption in the term 'embodiment' is that an individual's biology cannot be understood without considering the psychological, social and sociocultural aspects of development. An example of this is discrimination; there is evidence that the adverse effects of being discriminated against can get 'under the skin' of the individual and result in poor health. Embodiment relates to how we experience the world, and this includes our perceptions of our context and its possibilities, or its limits. Embodiment is affected by our experiences of illness, changes in our body image or ability to live our lives. Therefore an excessive emphasis on physiology and tests, whilst not recognising individuals within their wider social context, limits our ability to respond to another human being in a caring and dignified way.

Conclusion

As nursing students and qualified practitioners, maintaining the best standards of care in our area of practice is our individual and collective responsibility. Focusing care on what is important to individuals as human beings enables us as nurses to understand and more fully appreciate the individual's personal experience of ill health and therefore we can have a better understanding of how to support patients and promote their well-being. In doing so, this can ensure a patient-first approach to care which ensures we treat those we care for with respect and dignity.

Activities: brief outline answers

Activity 4.2

The way we care for patients on a one-to-one basis, and how we organise care overall, can make all the difference in whether those we care for have either a negative or positive experience. It is our responsibility to ensure that we always offer individual care, and organise care overall so the experience for those being cared for is positive.

Activity 4.4

You can give Jo choice wherever possible about when and where she eats and drinks, and what she eats and drinks; when she washes and which toilet she uses and how to get there safely; when she gets up and goes to bed, for instance. Encouraging and enabling Jo to make choices will help promote her well-being.

Activity 4.5

All the discussions you have had so far have been helping you to get to know Jo and helping you to build a relationship with her. You will need to discuss with Jo who she wants to have as contacts outside the hospital and who may be visiting or perhaps helping her on discharge and how much support they can offer.

Activity 4.6

All the dimensions of the humanising framework help to maintain dignity if used to help plan and inform care. They make sure that in putting Jo's experience at the heart of what you are doing, you are never causing distress or increasing suffering. This could be achieved through maintaining privacy, giving time to find out objects or tasks that give an individual comfort, flexibility about visiting times and always ensuring that we ask permission and offer explanations for everything we do as nurses.

Chapter 5
Physical aspects of ageing

Michele Board and Karen Cooper

NMC Standards for Pre-registration Nursing Education

Domain 3: Nursing practice and decision making

1. All nurses must use up-to-date knowledge and evidence to assess, plan, deliver and evaluate care, communicate findings, influence change and promote health and best practice. They must make person-centred, evidence-based judgments and decisions, in partnership with others involved in the care process, to ensure high quality care. They must be able to recognise when the complexity of clinical decisions requires specialist knowledge and expertise, and consult or refer accordingly.
3. All nurses must carry out comprehensive, systematic nursing assessments that take account of relevant physical, social, cultural, psychological, spiritual, genetic and environmental factors, in partnership with service users and others through interaction, observation and measurement.

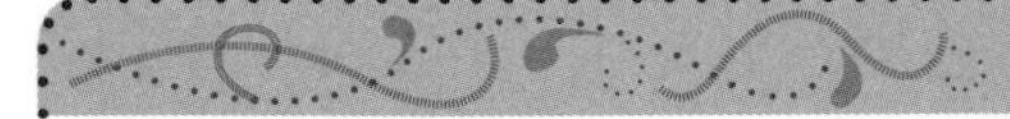

NMC Essential Skills Clusters (ESCs)

This chapter will support the following ESCs:

Care, compassion and communication

2. People can trust the newly registered graduate nurse to engage in person centred care empowering people to make choices about how their needs are met when they are unable to meet them for themselves.

2:2. Actively empowers people to be involved in the assessment and care planning process.

Organisational aspects of care

9. People can trust the newly registered graduate nurse to treat them as partners and work with them to make a holistic and systematic assessment of their needs; to develop a personalised plan that is based on mutual understanding and respect for their individual situation promoting health and well-being, minimising risk of harm and promoting their safety at all times.

9:9. Undertakes the assessment of physical, emotional, psychological, social, cultural and spiritual needs, including risk factors by working with the person and records, shares and responds to clear indicators and signs.

(continued)

continued ...

10. With the person and under supervision, plans safe and effective care by recording and sharing information based on the assessment.

By entry to the register

12. In partnership with the person, their carers and their families, makes a holistic, person centred and systematic assessment of physical, emotional, psychological, social, cultural and spiritual needs, including risk, and together, develops a comprehensive personalised plan of nursing care.
15. Works within the context of a multi-professional team and works collaboratively with other agencies when needed to enhance the care of people, communities and populations.
16. Promotes health and well-being, self care and independence by teaching and empowering people and carers to make choices in coping with the effects of treatment and the ongoing nature and likely consequences of a condition including death and dying.
19. Refers to specialists when required.

28. People can trust the newly qualified graduate nurse to assess and monitor their nutritional status and in partnership, formulate an effective plan of care.

28:1. Takes and records accurate measurements of weight, height, length, body mass index and other appropriate measures of nutritional status.

28:2. Assesses baseline nutritional requirements for healthy people related to factors such as age and mobility.

28:3. Contributes to formulating a care plan through assessment of dietary preferences, including local availability of foods and cooking facilities.

28:4. Reports to other members of the team when agreed plan is not achieved.

Medicines management

34. People can trust the newly registered graduate nurse to work within legal and ethical frameworks that underpin safe and effective medicines management.

34:4. Applies legislation to practice to safe and effective ordering, receiving, storing administering and disposal of medicines and drugs, including controlled drugs in both primary and secondary care settings and ensures others do the same.

35:4. Questions, critically appraises, takes into account ethical considerations and the preferences of the person receiving care and uses evidence to support an argument in determining when medicines may or may not be an appropriate choice of treatment.

36. People can trust the newly registered graduate nurse to ensure safe and effective practice in medicines management through comprehensive knowledge of medicines, their actions, risks and benefits.

36:1. Uses knowledge of commonly administered medicines in order to act promptly in cases where side effects and adverse reactions occur.

Chapter aims

On completion of this chapter you should be able to:

- understand how to complete a holistic assessment;
- appreciate the assessment of common physical needs of the older person.

Introduction

This chapter will focus on some of the more familiar physical problems encountered by people as they become older. Although we have been reluctant to adopt a biomedical model of individuals, we need a good grounding in anatomy and physiology to help people with problems of continence, confusion, falls, polypharmacy, nutrition and sensory impairment. In this chapter we will discuss your role as a nurse in assessing these needs.

Nursing assessment is an important and complex skill to acquire and develop throughout your nursing career. The aim of nursing assessment is to provide individualised and person-centred care according to the principles of the humanisation theory, discussed in Chapter 1.

In 2009 the Nursing and Midwifery Council (NMC) provided guidance on the nursing care of the older person, emphasising that adult nurses will inevitably spend much of their working time with older people. Here are some key facts from the NMC guidance, highlighting the significant number of older people in hospital and residential settings. Note they do emphasise that the majority of older people live independent lives with minimal or no assistance.

This means that all nurses must have some understanding of the nursing assessment and care of older people. A person may present with a familiar nursing need, such as nutrition, hydration or continence support, but how this manifests in an individual will be unique to each person. The appropriate use of nursing assessment skills will help identify and then plan how to meet these needs to suit the individual.

The NMC emphasises the importance of undertaking a comprehensive or holistic assessment, since an individual comes before the diagnosis. Nurses must avoid defining people as 'the dementia patient', or 'the stroke patient', where the diagnosis comes first and the person second.

Assessment is part of the nursing process, which is a cyclical system to help organise care delivery. Although not widely talked about now, the nursing process has four stages which will be familiar to all nurses. They are assessment, planning, implementation and evaluation. Planning of care will depend upon the wishes of the patients, the goals of care, as well as the available skill mix. The implementation of care must be evidence-based, with nurses knowing why and how they are implementing care in the way they are doing. The evaluation stage is when nurses and patients review how near they are to meeting the care goals. For example, has food intake increased, or is pain better controlled? The evaluation stage flows into a reassessment stage, where individual needs are reassessed and care plans reviewed once more. Assessment is not just undertaken once but is ongoing during that patient's journey.

Activity 5.1 — ***Case study***

Mr Alfred Wright, or Alf, as he likes to be called, is an 82-year-old man living in a residential setting. He has been living there for four months because his mobility was deteriorating and he was struggling to look after himself. His wife died two years before and he misses the breakfasts that she cooked and the way she attended to the small things that mattered, such as two sugars in his tea when he wakes up and bacon and eggs! Alf's mobility has deteriorated over the last four months. He appears less motivated to wash and dress and spends a lot of his time staring out of the window in his room. He joins the other residents for lunch but does not join in the social activities.

Questions to consider:

- You have been asked to undertake an assessment of Alf's needs. What do you need to consider?
- What skills do you need when undertaking an assessment?

As this is a personal reflection, no outline answer is supplied.

Outlined below is some guidance on nursing assessment.

Nursing assessment skills

Just by listening to Alf you will have already gleaned a great deal of information about his needs. Assessing Alf's needs takes a great deal of skill; we need to use effective communication skills. You will also need to take into account the normal effects of ageing, such as deterioration in hearing and vision, and ensure you speak clearly and also that your patient can see you clearly. Open questions allow people to tell you what is important to them, and what their care priorities are. An older person like Alf may hesitate as they speak, and talk slowly, but you need to give time to listen attentively.

A helpful guide to interviewing technique was devised by Egan (1975), who suggested an approach to ensure effective communication under the acronym SOLER:

S: Sit squarely, upright and alert.
O: Open posture: uncrossed arms and legs.
L: Lean forward, but not to the extent of invading their personal space.
E: Eye contact: maintain eye contact but do not stare.
R: Relax: this will demonstrate confidence.

Egan also reminds us of the importance of verbal and non-verbal communication. We need to observe patients' non-verbal cues when we are assessing them. Do they look agitated or in pain? Patients too will be observing your non-verbal cues: do you look interested in what they are saying? To facilitate verbal interaction you could incorporate the appropriate use of open and closed questions, reflecting, paraphrasing, echoing and summarising in your assessments. Non-verbally, you could respond to people through postural echo, nodding, smiling, touch and silence, all of which are powerful when used at the right time. Stickley also included touch and intuition. *Respectful use of touch can communicate compassion, love, empathy and understanding* (Krieger, 1990, cited by Stickley, 2011). Benner (1984) discusses the important role intuition plays when assessing and caring for people.

Holistic assessment

When assessing Alf a holistic perspective, as outlined by the NMC, and presented in Figure 5.1, can be used as a guide.

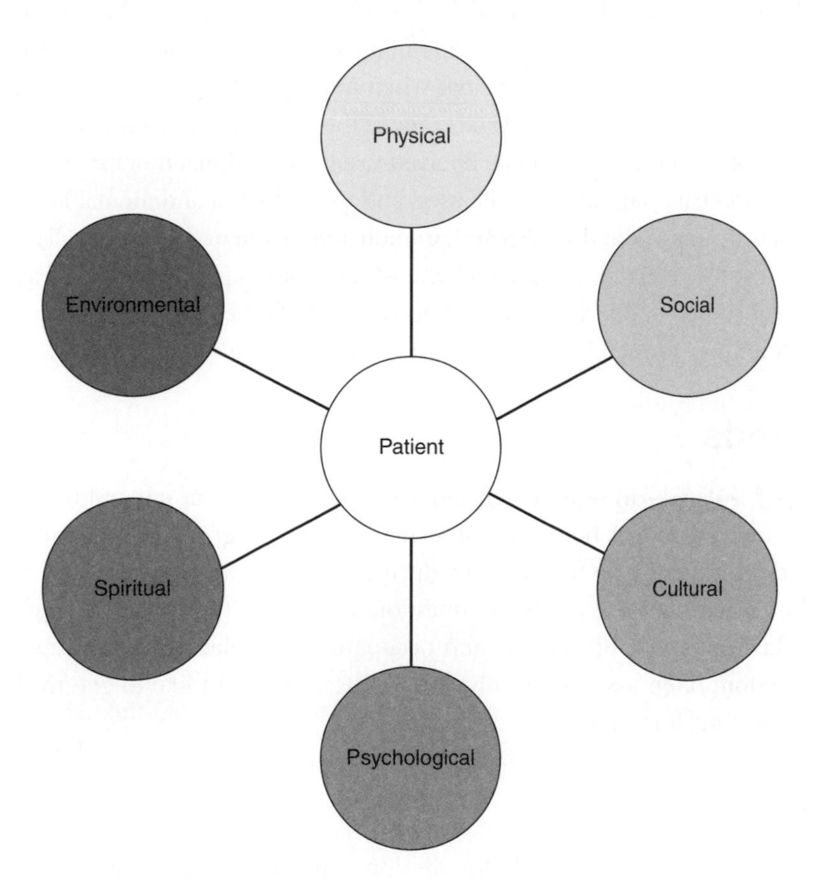

Figure 5.1: A model for holistic assessment

Physical needs

The NMC definition and Figure 5.1 remind us that the whole is greater than the sum of its parts. Nevertheless a physical assessment of your patient's needs is essential. Identifying what assistance Alf needs with his activities of daily living is a helpful start. It is important to establish what Alf can do for himself and encourage his independence. Alf mentions that when he arrived at the care home he was able to walk with a frame, but since his arrival his mobility has deteriorated and he now feels embarrassed because he needs assistance to go to the toilet. You would need to ask Alf to clarify, but it appears he now has a catheter, when he says, 'Sometimes you know it gets too full and then it pulls'. Two key issues emerge from this: why Alf's mobility has deteriorated and why he has a catheter in situ (see later for continence assessment). You will also need to consider why Alf's mobility has deteriorated. Is there a physical reason, such as pain, or have his muscles started to weaken because he has not been encouraged to mobilise and exercise as he was doing before? For expediency we must avoid using a wheelchair when a person is able to walk, albeit slowly. Muscle mass decreases with age and therefore exercising to maintain muscle strength is crucial (Knight and Nigam, 2008b). We can 'care to death' by doing too much for an individual and not only remove patients' autonomy, but also their independence.

Poor nutrition will lead to deterioration in health (see nutritional assessment, later). So identifying Alf's personal preferences for diet is essential. This is important since it will make Alf feel that his likes and dislikes will be taken into account; attending to the small things such as how he likes his tea will increase his self-esteem and well-being. When nursing older people team work is essential. Effective team working is an essential skill and is one of the pleasures when looking after people with complex needs. For example, Alf could be referred to an occupational therapist whatever care setting he is in. An occupational therapist will assess and treat physical and mental health conditions using specific activity to prevent disability and promote independent function in all aspects of daily life. Alf should also be referred to a physiotherapist. Physiotherapists help and treat people with physical problems caused by illness, accident or ageing. A physiotherapist will provide an assessment of Alf's mobility and recommend exercises to sustain or improve his independence.

Social needs

Being lonely and isolated can significantly impact upon our sense of self and well-being in later life. Humans are social beings; being part of society and a social group can validate personhood. Assessing what older people do to keep busy during the day, how they like to spend their time, and what hobbies they have, are important questions to ask, and then act upon, regardless of the care setting. Having a sense of purpose and occupation each day will improve self-worth and relieve the boredom often associated with care settings. Alf might like to get involved in some gardening or painting, for example.

Cultural needs

Culture is often defined as the 'way things are done around here'. When we speak about the cultural needs of an individual, we mean the ways we express ourselves as humans, which could relate to religion, gender roles, social conventions or social norms – all of which vary in different age groups. For example, as an older person Alf may have experienced different social norms to a younger person. He and his wife may have adopted specific gender roles in their family, with his wife undertaking the meal preparation and running of the home, and Alf perhaps going out to work. As nurses we must therefore be aware of this if the health of one of the couple deteriorates, since we may need to support the couple to adapt and undertake new roles. For example, Alf discusses how his wife cooked him a lovely breakfast each day. She may have prepared all the meals. Many older men say that until they were widowed they 'couldn't even boil an egg'. In a care setting, an appreciation of an individual's life history is essential, to enable the team to encourage continued social engagement, by undertaking activities that an individual has previously undertaken. We should be aware of the different gender needs. For example, the men in a residential setting will be a minority group, since women do live longer. As a group the men may prefer a different set of activities from the women, and consideration should be given to this.

Care delivery is also affected by the culture of the care setting; the accepted norms and practices in the home may not encourage independence of thought or activity. Kitwood (1997) refers to the *malignant social psychology* of a social environment in which interactions and communications occur which diminish the 'personhood' of people experiencing it. People whose uniqueness is not recognised can 'shrink' and feel less human.

Activity 5.2 *Reflection*

- When you have or have had a placement in a residential setting what activities were the residents encouraged to participate in?
- Did these activities have a gender bias?
- What activities do you think different genders might specifically enjoy?

An outline answer is provided at the end of the chapter.

Psychological needs

Sense of self has been identified as an important feature of well-being in older people. Sense of self is shown in the way we present ourselves – our dress style, for instance – as well as our interactions with others. Here are some ways we can help individuals to retain their sense of self.

- Ensure people are asked how they would like to be addressed and that staff respect this.
- Avoid negative labels to define people, e.g. 'bed blockers', 'doubles', 'feeds', 'wanderer'.
- Allow people to choose what they would like to wear.
- Ensure people are given all the information on the service, in the appropriate format and, wherever possible, in advance.
- Care planning should include opportunities for patients to talk with staff regularly.
- Involve people in the production of information resources.
- Facilitate ways of getting the views of patients, such as through residents' meetings.

Woolhead et al. (2004) sought the views of older people about dignity, who remarked how inferior they feel in comparison with the healthcare professional, noting:

> *Patients don't possess the health and vigour or knowledge of those looking after them, which means that they're in an unequal situation. In fact, they're in a position of decided inferiority with regard to health, vigour and knowledge.*

As nurses we need to work towards an inclusive relationship with patients to enable them to retain their sense of self.

Spiritual needs

Spirituality is a significant dimension of well-being.

> *Holistic care, based on the premises that there is a balance between body, mind and spirit, is important for well-being, that each of these is interconnected, and that each affects the others. Human spirit is considered to be the essence of being and is what motivates and guides us to live a meaningful existence.*
> (Narayanasamy et al., 2004)

Spiritual needs, if expressed outside a religious framework, are very likely to go unnoticed. Allowing and facilitating discussions with older people around their sense of meaning, and their life's purpose, requires space, time and respect for their privacy and dignity.

Environmental needs

Assessment of older people's environment involves asking them about their current living arrangements. See Table 5.1 for questions to inform your assessment.

Information you need to collect	Relevance
Who do they live with?	An older person living alone without any form of support is more likely to be admitted to a residential setting
	Living with a partner/family support/good neighbours can provide support with increasing age
	Assistance with shopping, heavy housework and gardening enables the older person to remain independent
	Having people drop in regularly enables older people to retain social contact, as with increasing age their world shrinks (Biley et al., 2011)
Where do they live?	It is important to know whether a person lives in a house, bungalow, flat, assisted living or residential setting. Access in and out of the property and quality of housing can be assessed by an occupational therapist, who will be able to identify if any modifications or aids need to be undertaken or supplied to enable older people to remain independent and in their own home if they wish
How do they prepare meals, including shopping?	Access to shops and preparation of meals will give an indication of the older person's ability to have a balanced diet
How do they access the toilet, during the day and night? Access to the bath/shower	Does the older person have easy access to the toilet during the day and night? Is the lighting appropriate, is the bathroom warm? Is access always up and down stairs? If so, can the older person negotiate these safely?

Table 5.1: Assessment of the living environment

Living in a residential setting should look and feel like home. Staff working in these areas will have an excellent opportunity to work with individual clients to make them feel at home. You might like to think what makes you feel at home. It could be the sense of control you feel about who enters your home. It could be the relationships you have with the people you live with or who visit your home. It could be having your favourite things around you, such as photographs, books, a favourite chair. Having your own bed with your favourite linen and being able to bathe when you want are all features that could make you feel 'at home'. Home is a place of sensory satisfaction. The sound of the house, the feel of the textures under your hands and feet, access to your favourite foods, seeing your life displayed around you, and sharing that with others are often considered as important aspects of the meaning of home.

Assessment of people with acute confusion or delirium

Whatever care setting you work in, you will work with older patients who appear confused and disoriented. The concern is that this confusion will be considered a normal part of ageing and not be assessed, and the cause for the confusion not identified. *The human brain has so many neurons that it has a natural built-in redundancy that allows it to adequately cope with the physical changes that are associated with ageing* (Knight and Nigam, 2008a, p. 18). There are many reasons why older people may be confused; they may be depressed, have dementia or have a delirium, a mixture, or even all of these.

For further information about differential diagnosis and dementia, see Barker and Board (2012).

Activity 5.3 — *Reflection*

Think of a time when you have looked after someone who appeared confused. What was the person saying or doing that made you think the individual was confused? There may even be a time when you yourself felt confused, perhaps coming round after an anaesthetic, and if so, what did it feel like?

With a colleague, discuss and list reasons that might cause confusion in an older adult.

An outline answer is given at the end of the chapter.

When individuals are confused they can appear disoriented to time and place. They may not know where they are, what time it is or where they are if they are in a care environment. They may struggle to maintain their attention on the conversation or recall things that you have said. They can appear muddled and may be distressed or even quite cheerful. They may be agitated or very quiet. As you can imagine, they may feel very afraid. However it is crucial that staff assess the mental or cognitive state of all their patients, particularly older patients. The confusion assessment tool is a quick tool used by nurses which indicates whether a more comprehensive assessment is required.

Confusion assessment

The confusion assessment tool is a quick tool used in identifying confusion. A comprehensive nursing assessment is indicated if features 1 and 2 and 3 or 4 in the list are present:

1. acute onset and fluctuating course;
2. inattention;
3. disorganised thinking;
4. altered level of consciousness.

Acute onset of confusion is likely to be caused by a delirium. As with all alterations in cognition, a comprehensive assessment is needed. Acute confusion or delirium is characterised by disorganised thinking, a decreased attention span and fluctuating consciousness, disturbance in the sleep–wake cycle, disorientation and changes in psychomotor skills (Henry, 2002). Acute confusion caused by a delirium is different from dementia or depression because its onset is more rapid.

The risk of morbidity (dying) from delirium increases from between 22 and 76 per cent when the cause is undiagnosed. The length of stay in hospital is likely to increase, as are the chances of developing pressure ulcers, falls, pneumonia and hospital-acquired infections. Those who survive undiagnosed delirium are more likely to be transferred to long-term care with a decline in both functional and cognitive status. This has a subsequent financial cost for both health and social care providers (Barker and Board, 2012).

The charity Age Concern launched a campaign in 2007 to raise awareness of the assessment and management of delirium. They emphasised that acute confusion is a sign that someone is physically unwell. They identify a three-point plan for the assessment and management of delirium: Spot it, Treat it and Stop it.

Spotting delirium can be a challenge. The literature identifies three types of delirium: hyperactive, hypoactive and mixed. Hyperactive delirium is characterised by restlessness, agitation and irritability and may include hallucinations. In contrast, the hypoactive form manifests as withdrawal, apathy, lethargy and decreased psychomotor activity. This latter form is difficult to recognise because the person may be assumed to be compliant and contented. Fluctuations can also occur between hyperactivity and hypoactivity (Barker and Board, 2012).

The acronym PINCH ME provides a useful *aide-mémoire* when assessing the cause of an acute confusion. Assessment for these signs will help identify the most common causes of delirium: Pain, INfection, Constipation, Hydration, Medication, Environment.

Pain

If you have ever experienced pain, such as a broken arm or childbirth, you know that it can cause momentary lapses in concentration and organised thinking. When older people experience pain they can have prolonged periods of disorientation and confusion. Their inability to express this may well be influenced by a history of stoicism, whereby they believe they should learn to cope with pain.

Pain can cause disorientation and confusion. The Abbey pain scale is useful for assessing pain in a confused patient (Royal College of Physicians, 2007). This scale involves assessment of:

- vocalisations – such as crying;
- facial expression – such as grimacing;
- change of body language – such as holding parts of the body;
- behavioural change – such as refusing to eat;
- physiological change – such as blood pressure;
- physical changes – such as skin tears.

Equally important is reassessment of the patient after medications have been administered to ensure pain is mitigated (Phillips, 2013).

Infection

Nurses play a crucial role in the identification and treatment of infection, because of their close relationship with patients. The treatment and management of infection are essential to prevent further deterioration of health.

Activity 5.4 — ***Critical thinking***

First make a list of assessment activities you can undertake to identify an infection.

How would you report your findings?

An outline answer is provided at the end of the chapter.

Constipation

Impacted hard faeces or the passing of small hard stools is constipation. With increasing age, peristalsis slows, increasing the transit time of waste in the large intestine, which can lead to constipation (Nigam and Knight, 2008a). Regular recording of bowel actions whilst in a care environment is essential since a new environment can increase the risk of becoming constipated.

Hydration

Dehydration is more common in old age because renal function is reduced. The ability of the kidneys to maintain homeostasis decreases with age, so that by the age of 80 a person's renal function is half of what it was when that person was 40 (Andrade and Knight, 2008). Older people are more susceptible to vascular diseases as they age, which can lead to chronic conditions that affect the renal system, such as diabetes. This is compounded by the fact that, even when dehydrated, older people experience a diminished sense of thirst and a lack of desire to drink. If prescribed diuretics that increase urine output an older person may reduce fluid intake to avoid going to the toilet too much.

Medication review

It is important to record all the medication that patients are taking. Polypharmacy and certain medications such as antidepressants or opiates can cause confusion. Therefore the medical team will need to review these as part of the multidimensional assessment. See later section on medication assessment.

Environment

There is some evidence to suggest that sensory deprivation experienced by patients placed in windowless hospital rooms is associated with higher rates of delirium. These potentially modifiable risk factors include multiple room/ward changes, use of medical or physical restraints, and absence of a clock, watch or reading glasses, hearing aid not used and lack of familiar faces/objects (McCusker et al., 2001).

Continence assessment

Continence is a major issue affecting older people. It is estimated that 20 per cent of older people living in their own homes and 30–60 per cent of older people in long-term care experience issues with incontinence (Wagg et al., 2008). Incontinence can also be a major stressor on carers who are caring for a loved one at home, and can contribute to decisions regarding whether to place the individual in a care home. Incontinence can include both urinary and faecal, yet urinary incontinence is more prevalent and as such it shall be the type of incontinence focused upon.

That said, there are normal ageing processes which impact upon continence in older people. As we age, the neurological pathways between bladder and brain become less sensitive and as a result older people are not aware that they need to go to the toilet until their bladder is 90 per cent full, compared to younger adults, whose bladders register the need to go to the toilet when they are 50 per cent full (Nazarko, 2008). This is really important to remember as when older people say they need to go to the toilet, they do; their ability to wait is reduced in comparison to younger people.

Activity 5.5 *Reflection*

Think about how you would feel if you were unable to get to the toilet in time and as a consequence experienced urinary incontinence. Write a list of words or a sentence to describe your feelings.

As this is a personal reflection, no outline answer is supplied.

In this activity you may have listed words such as shame, anxiety, embarrassment, distress, yet often we as nurses forget that people can feel like this. Going to the toilet is normally a very private affair for the majority of our lives and many of us are not used to emptying our bladder in front of someone else. Older people experience the same emotions and feelings regarding incontinence that you also feel and urinary incontinence can be very distressing for older people, resulting in them becoming depressed and socially isolated. Therefore any discussion with older people must be handled tactfully and sensitively – think about how you would feel if a stranger asked you about your toilet habits.

Assessment

Even though incontinence can be reversible (Table 5.2), whether or not people access services and treatment is largely dependent upon the attitude of the care staff. Older people who seek help for their concerns and worries regarding incontinence often receive poor-quality continence care (Nazarko, 2008). As nurses we tend to focus upon managing the incontinence through the use of pads, rather than undertaking a systematic continence assessment. A comprehensive continence assessment would include:

- History – finding out the exact details of the problems the individual is having with regard to continence.
- Investigation – finding out fluid intake and output as well as the numbers and timings of any episodes of incontinence. The use of a bladder diary over three days is really useful here to get a full picture regarding the nature of their difficulties.
- Physical examination – this needs to be undertaken by a trained nurse who has undergone additional skills and education. This can identify any abnormalities present and should also include a rectal examination.
- Assessment of activities of daily living – assessing the individual's ability to undertake activities of living as well as any difficulties the person is experiencing, as this may highlight difficulties with removing clothing which can impact upon continence.
- Medication – assessing whether any of the client's current medication could be impacting on continence.

(adapted from Nazarko, 2008)

D: Delirium

I: Infection (urinary tract infection)

A: Atrophy (urogenital atrophy in women)

P: Psychological (depression)

P: Pharmacological (medication)

E: Excess urine output

R: Restricted mobility

S: Stool impactions (constipation)

(Geriatric Medicine and Nursing Standard, 2008)

Table 5.2: Reversible causes of urinary incontinence

Types of urinary incontinence

There are many different types of urinary incontinence and identifying the type is paramount if we are to treat or manage it effectively. Table 5.3 details the different types of urinary incontinence as well as identifying the common symptoms.

Stress: Leaking urine when your bladder is under pressure, such as laughing, sneezing, coughing or undertaking strenuous activity
Urge: A sudden and urgent need to pass urine when you are unable to delay, often just having a few seconds before the desire to urinate and actually urinating. Getting up several times during the night to urinate
Mixed: Less common but includes a mixture of both stress and urge incontinence
Overflow incontinence: More common in men who have an enlarged prostate – this is where you pass small trickles of urine very often and your bladder still feels full after you have been to the toilet
Overactive bladder syndrome: Similar to urge, as you have a frequent and urgent need to urinate, yet you may not actually experience being incontinent

Table 5.3: Types of urinary incontinence and common symptoms

Treatment for incontinence is multifaceted and this is why a thorough assessment is required. Treatments can include pelvic floor therapy, drug therapy and surgery. In pelvic floor therapy, individuals are taught how to strengthen their pelvic floor. This is achieved by asking people to squeeze their pelvic floor (imagine you need to break wind but are desperately trying to hold it in) and as such undertaking these exercises can strengthen the pelvic floor. You need to do this 10–15 times in a row on a daily basis. However, many people struggle to locate their pelvic floor and sometimes things like weighted vaginal cones can assist.

Drug therapy is also used; specific medications are available to assist with urinary incontinence which can be considered.

Surgery is also available; there are a number of surgical treatments to treat urinary incontinence.

In addition to this, there are of course containment treatments such as the use of incontinence products (such as pads) and catheters and convenes. A thorough assessment is at the heart of finding the right treatment for the individual. Other recommendations can include examining what the person is drinking and at what time of night (for example, drinking caffeine should be avoided, especially late at night). Part of the management of continence is enabling people to go to the toilet, especially if they require assistance. We as nurses need to examine how we enable people to go to the toilet, and the degree to which we offer privacy. You need to ask yourself whether you would be happy to use a commode behind a curtain or whether you would be able to use the toilet you are offering patients. If the answer is no, then should we expect patients to do it? It is vital that when we are assisting people to go to the toilet we try to remember how it feels rather than simply thinking 'we are toileting them', as this reduces this highly private aspect of personal care to a mundane and routine chore.

Nutritional assessment

The importance of nutrition and fluid management was discussed in Chapter 2. This chapter will focus on the assessment of these needs and actions. Ensuring that the nutritional needs are met is part of the nurse's role and a requirement for meeting the ESC.

> *It is a national scandal that six out of 10 older people are at risk of becoming malnourished, or their situation getting worse, in hospital. Ending the scandal of malnourished older people in hospitals will save lives.*
> (Age Concern, 2006)

This is a quote from the *Hungry to be Heard* report, which also included feedback from older people and their relatives about the nutritional care they received. Rather than things improving, Age UK (2010b) discusses that, if anything, they have got worse.

Case study

Joan, 83 years old, was admitted to hospital following an accident at home. Prior to admission, she had lost 6 lb in a week and her family were concerned about the weight loss. During her third week in hospital, Joan lost 10 lb in weight. Her son, Bernard, was concerned about the help with eating that his mother was receiving – a concern shared by fellow visitors. The hospital had a sign saying, 'If you feel that your relatives need assistance during mealtimes, you are welcome to come in and assist us'. However, Bernard couldn't always be there at mealtimes as he was busy trying to find a care home for his mother. Bernard could not understand why his mother's weight loss was being recorded but nothing done to help her eat.

Activity 5.6 — *Reflection*

Read the case study above, which is one of the extracts from the Age Concern report.

Reflect on this case study and what you have experienced within your practice placements. Note down any areas of good practice, such as protected mealtimes; any coloured tray policies; regular charting; environment; and staff taking time.

As this is a personal reflection, no outline answer is supplied.

Food and water are essential for life and when we are unwell we need to eat the right food, in the right amounts and at the right time. Nutritional assessment is an ongoing process that will provide key information to help you plan and evaluate the care given. Food, and help with eating it, should be recognised by ward staff as important in showing respect for the dignity of older people. Help with eating should be readily given and be seen as a priority. Dehumanising terms such as 'how many feeders' and 'having to feed' should not be used.

Fletcher (2009) stresses the importance of nursing nutritional assessment, taking into account a patient's overall clinical, physical and psychological condition, including factors that may affect appetite (Best and Evans, 2013). You need to assess the following physical areas: the patient's usual weight; body mass index (BMI); changes in appetite, taste, smell, chewing, swallowing; past medical history and recent medical history, such as any surgery, infection or trauma; any diarrhoea and vomiting; and medications and alcohol consumption. In terms of observational assessment, look at the patient's normal weight, and distribution of weight; whether clothing or jewellery is loose-fitting, especially rings; dentures, which if loose-fitting could indicate recent weight loss and will impact on the patient's ability to eat; skin conditions, such as dry skin or reduced elasticity, which may indicate dehydration or a poor protein intake; oral condition, for example, what is the condition of the tongue?; any bleeding of the gums and condition of the teeth. Evidence of sores at the corner of the mouth or a sore tongue can indicate a vitamin B deficiency, food allergies or intolerance.

You will also need to assess psychosocial factors:

- living arrangements, who the patient lives with and location;
- recent bereavement: a recent bereavement may reduce appetite;
- shopping and cooking: being unable to shop or cook may impact on the choice of food and would also need to be taken into account for early effective discharge planning;
- environment during mealtimes;
- eating patterns: whether the patient can eat independently;
- cognition.

Screening should assess BMI and percentage unintentional weight loss over a specific time period. A person is malnourished as indicated by any of the following:

- BMI of less than 18.5 kg/m^2;
- unintentional weight loss greater than 10 per cent within the last three to six months;
- BMI of less than 20 kg/m^2 and unintentional weight loss greater than 5 per cent within the last three to six months.

(National Institute for Health and Care Excellence (NICE), 2006)

It is important that you not only undertake nutritional screening, as recommended by NICE (2006), but also act on the results. In the case study on Joan, it would appear that assessments were undertaken but the family were not aware of any planned actions following the assessment, such as referral to a dietician, regular weight reassessments and monitoring of food and fluid intake. This should include food and fluid charts, daily or weekly weight, regular BMI and use of a screening tool such as the Malnutrition Universal Screening Tool (MUST). MUST is a simple, validated tool developed by the British Association of Parental and Enteral

Nutrition (BAPEN) and is used to screen for the risk of malnutrition. The Department of Health (2010c) *Essence of Care* benchmark on nutrition supports the need for full assessment of individuals' nutritional status along with ensuring that they and their carers are involved in decisions.

Medicine management

Refer back to Chapter 2 if necessary, where we discussed the importance of medicine management. As we are an ageing society, living longer with complex, chronic illness, the number of medications we take as we age and experience comorbidity increases. Yet the Department of Health (2001a) identifies that as many as 50 per cent of older people may not be taking medicines as they have been prescribed, resulting in a waste of about £100 million a year. We have all seen patients at home or even relatives with bags of unused medications. What contributes to this problem?

NICE identifies two main reasons why older people do not take their medicines: it may be intentional, where the patient makes a conscious decision not to take a medicine, and this may be due to side-effects or being unhappy with the prescribed regime. It may be unintentional, where patients are happy to take the prescribed medication but experience difficulties in doing so. These difficulties may be linked to issues with physical dexterity, poor memory and/or confusion or simply forgetting to take the medication.

How do we as nurses know whether patients are intentionally or unintentionally not complying with medicine regimes? It is really important here to assess older people upon admission to hospital or within their own home to develop an understanding of if and how they take their medication. It is vital that this assessment is undertaken in a non-judgemental capacity; rather it is simply a fact-finding mission. Key questions (adapted from Peate, 2003) that can be used by nurses to assess patients' understanding and knowledge of their medicine regimes include:

- How long have you been taking this medication?
- Is it in its original container?
- Why are you taking this?
- Do you know how often and when?
- Do you have a daily routine for taking your medicine?
- Do you experience any difficulties?
- Do you experience any side-effects?
- Do you have any allergies?
- Do you take any over-the-counter medication?
- Do you take any vitamins, herbal or homeopathic remedies?
- Do you use any other form of medicines – prescribed or not?

If you identify as part of this assessment that a patient has been intentionally choosing not to take medication, our role is not to criticise. We have to remember that, under the Mental Capacity Act, older people with capacity are entitled to make decisions regarding their own life and are therefore free to choose not to undergo medication treatment for a health condition and this has to be respected. Our role in this circumstance is to ensure that patients are making an informed choice by providing information and then respecting the decision they make. It is also really important that older people are involved in decisions regarding any new medication being prescribed.

If the assessment identifies that patients have been unintentionally not taking their medication because of difficulties, then our role is to work with patients and their family (if appropriate) to assist them in developing strategies to support them with their medication regime. It is important that medication is prescribed in a way that fits with the patient's lifestyle with minimal need for prompts, such as once or twice a day. We need to encourage patients to associate taking their medication with key points of the day – such as with breakfast, or the morning cup of tea. This then encourages developing a sense of routine with taking medication which can increase compliance. We also can explore whether a compliance aid would be useful for the older person.

Multicompartment compliance aids are boxes in which a person's medication can be added and then it reminds them during the day to take these. Compliance aids can be a daily aid filled by the patient or family or a weekly box filled by the community pharmacist. It is important to note that compliance aids have both advantages and disadvantages (Table 5.4) and as such they do not suit every patient, which is why an individual assessment of needs is fundamental. The most important issue for older people was remaining in control and being independent and therefore making decisions for older people without their knowledge removes this sense of control (Nunney et al., 2011).

Advantages	**Disadvantages**
Acts as a visual prompt to remind patient/carers that the medicine needs to be taken or has been taken	Patient and/or carers must be educated regarding how to use the device Can only be used for tablets
Acts as a memory aid	Not suitable for PRN (as required medication), only suitable for tablets
Provides reassurance as it is sealed	Not suitable if frequent adjustments are required
Can help manage complex regimes	Usually only has four spaces a day
Supports care agencies to administer medicines	Difficult to identify individual tables
Can be labelled to identify the medicines contained in the device	Requires physical dexterity to open the pack and retrieve the tablets
Protects against moisture and contamination once the device is sealed	Limited space
	Filling the device is time-consuming and costly

Table 5.4: Advantages and disadvantages of a monitored dosage system

(Source: adapted from Emblin, 2011)

It is also vital that, at the point of discharge, we as nurses spend time with older people explaining their medication to them, ensuring that they and their family (if appropriate) are correctly educated regarding the use and storage and how and when to take their medication. Remember that many of the advice labels on the packets are simply too small for older people to read and as such it is good practice to write out a list of the medications and administration guidelines as well as any common side-effects.

Sensory impairment

Impaired vision and hearing are common among older adults. Loss of these senses increases the risk of depression, falls and suicide, and cognitive decline is exacerbated (Cupples, 2012). Deteriorating sight impacts upon independence and well-being and reduces quality of life. Age-related hearing loss, however, is more frequent and is associated with an increased risk of depression, and impairs quality of life and the ability to conduct activities of daily living, as well as leading to an increased reliance on community and informal supports (Gopinath et al., 2013). Wearing glasses is perceived to be more socially acceptable, whereas the use of hearing aids is less acceptable, with people feeling that hearing aids display their ageing more overtly than wearing glasses.

The ear perceives sounds and maintains balance. With normal ageing hearing deteriorates. The rate of hearing loss can be increased with exposure to loud noises during working life or leisure pursuits (i.e. factories, road works, musicians), especially if ear protection muffs have not been worn. Hearing loss is termed presbycusis. The mechanisms of the ear become less able to hear sounds at high frequencies, which typifies presbycusis. There can also be a build-up of cerumen (wax) within the ear, mainly because it becomes drier because there is a reduction in the production of sweat with age. Also with ageing the ear's ability to help maintain balance is reduced, increasing the risk of dizziness and reducing balance (Nigam and Knight, 2008b).

Scenario

Mr Jones is a 75-year-old married man. He lives in a semidetached house with his wife. He is completely independent. He wears glasses for reading and driving and has, according to his wife, 'gone deaf'; she says that she needs to keep repeating herself because he ignores her.

Activity 5.7 — *Decision making*

In light of Mr Jones's sensory loss, what should you take into consideration during the assessment process, admission into hospital, subsequent surgery and recovery before discharge home?

An outline answer is provided at the end of the chapter.

Tables 5.5 and 5.6 outline nursing considerations for communicating with people with visual impairment and those who are hard of hearing.

- When communicating, the following might be appropriate: letters in large print, with different font styles, or with background contrast, or offering information in audio format, by telephone or electronically (e-mail or compact disc), rather than letter. Braille letters or information could be needed
- Give an initial greeting as you enter the patient's room/bed space, explain what you are doing and how, and check this is understood before starting care interventions
- Describe the room layout, the other people who are in the room and what is happening
- Try to avoid situations where competing background noise may be a problem
- People with visual impairment may require simple clear instructions or personal physical guidance to find their way around
- Offer assistance, your arm, for example, for guidance
- Use accurate and specific language when giving directions. For example, 'the toilet is on your left'
- Explain surfaces/steps
- Explain when and how to access food and drink, and when meals are served; explain location, use the clock face to help, e.g. meat at 3 o'clock
- Never guide someone into a seat backwards: instead, describe the chair, place your hand on the back of the chair, and enable the person to orientate him- or herself into the seat independently
- Use whatever vision remains
- Ask how you may help: increasing the light, reading the menu, describing where things are, where it is best for you to stand/sit when communicating
- Treat people in the same respectful way regardless of the impairment
- With regard to patients' visual impairment, they are the expert, so check with them what further support or guidance they would prefer

Table 5.5: Nursing considerations: impact of poor vision in hospital

(Source: adapted from Cupples, 2012)

- If the person wears a hearing aid and still has difficulty hearing, check to see if the hearing aid is in the person's ear. Check to see that it is turned on, adjusted and has a working battery
- Get the attention of the person who is hard of hearing before you start to speak, to enable the individual to use all the non-verbal forms of communication, such as lip reading, facial expressions and body language
- Speak at your normal volume, and slightly more slowly. Do not shout or exaggerate your lip patterns as this will distort the message. Lack of clarity of speech sounds is often more of a problem than lack of volume
- Don't eat or chew when you are communicating

- Keep your hands away from your face while talking; do not turn away or undertake other actions such as pulling the curtains when communicating; make sure the patient can see your face at all times
- Recognise that hard-of-hearing people hear and understand less well when they are tired or ill
- Reduce or eliminate background noise as far as possible when carrying on conversations. Soft furnishings will absorb noise and reduce echo
- Use simple, short sentences to make your conversation easier to understand
- Write messages if necessary
- Allow ample time to converse with a hearing-impaired person. Being in a rush will compound everyone's stress and create barriers to a meaningful conversation

Table 5.6: Nursing considerations: communicating with the hearing-impaired

(Source: information from Deaf Action: **http://www.deafaction.org**)

Falls

Falls and related injuries are a significant problem for both health and social care services and have a profound impact on the person's quality of life and well-being (Barker, 2013). Every year, more than one in three – 3.4 million people – over 65 suffer a fall that can cause serious injury, and even death (Age UK, 2012). There has recently been a revised NICE clinical guideline (2013). This offers practical advice on the care of older people who are at risk of falling. Falls assessment must address individual factors and work to reduce these risks.

Case study

Mary is an 87-year-old woman who lives alone in a bungalow, where she has lived for the past eight years. She was widowed over 20 years ago but has a son who lives away and a daughter locally. Her daughter has cerebral palsy and is wheelchair-dependent and stays with her mother at the weekends. Mary does her own shopping and cooking but has a cleaner and a private gardener. She enjoys 'pottering' in her garden, weeding and potting plants. She walks with a stick when she goes outside but not in the bungalow. She wears glasses for reading and her short-term memory is poor. She takes aspirin and antihypertensive medication which she has been prescribed for a number of years. Mary has recently had a hospital admission, having fallen in the garden, where she sustained skin lacerations but no bony injury. She has been anxious since her discharge home about future falls and has been reluctant to go out as often as she had done before.

Activity 5.8 — *Decision making*

Make a list of the factors that you may need to consider in assessing Mary and the risk of falling.

As this is a personal reflection, no outline answer is supplied.

You may have listed several factors, including medication, and whether her blood pressure is low; her environment and whether there are any obstacles such as the stability of furniture, steps and type of flooring, along with her visual ability; her gait and balance, along with recognising her normal routine and any aids that help.

Risk factors for falls

The World Health Organization (2007c) proposed this risk factor model for falls in older age:

- behavioural: medication; alcohol; lack of exercise; inappropriate footwear;
- environment: poor building design; slippery floors and stairs; loose rugs; insufficient lighting; cracked or uneven pavements or sidewalks;
- biological: age and gender; chronic illness; arthritis; osteoporosis; physical and cognitive decline;
- socioeconomic: low income; inadequate housing; lack of social interactions; lack of community resources.

The multiprofessional team

The team members may include a dietician, as a good nutritional intake will help with stamina and exercise. A podiatrist will check foot and nail condition and give advice on footwear, e.g. insoles. An occupational therapist will assess the environment and advise on any appropriate aids and adaptations, home assessment and safety modifications. A physiotherapist may give foot and ankle exercises, balance exercises and fall prevention advice. The GP may review medication, the optician check vision and social services give support and financial advice.

Assessment for falls

Gillespie et al. (2012) and Nyman et al. (2011) also highlighted the need for health professionals to recognise that many people do not acknowledge falls because of negative stereotyping, the belief that falls are inevitable in older age and embarrassment about losing control. NICE has set key priorities for implementation, one of which is: *Older people who present for medical attention because of a fall, or report recurrent falls in the past year, or demonstrate abnormalities of gait and/or balance should be offered a multifactorial falls risk assessment* (NICE, 2013, p. 7).

Such an assessment should include: identification of falls history, cardiovascular examination and medication review; assessment of gait, balance and mobility, and muscle weakness; osteoporosis risk; perceived functional ability and fear relating to falling; visual impairment; cognitive impairment and neurological examination; urinary incontinence and home hazards.

NICE (2013) provides a quick reference guide regarding falls assessment and prevention which could be used as a checklist in the practice environment. There are also many falls assessment tools available; for example, the Morse Falls scale, STRATIFY tool and the falls risk assessment tool (FRAT) are just some that are commonly used and you should ask about these during your clinical placements.

Oliver and Healey (2009) identify that it is important to recognise that some patients who are at high risk will not fall and others may fall who score as a low risk. Assessing the person's fear and anxiety linked to falls requires effective communication skills to support decisions within a trusting, therapeutic relationship. Hadjistavropoulos et al. (2011) discussed the impact of the fear and anxiety associated with falling as a downward spiral. Avoiding activity leads to muscle decline and instability, which increase the risk of future falls. Many older people do not injure themselves in a fall, but have great difficulty getting up again afterwards and may stay on the floor for some time, and lack of physical fitness is now acknowledged as a key factor. Physical exercise not only improves muscle strength but also improves mental health and well-being. Age Concern (2012) recommends activities twice a week, and these can include gardening and dancing and should include balance training. The nurse needs to explore why people may not exercise, for example, not being fully aware of the benefits or lack of facilities or transport. During your practice placements identify what exercise groups and falls prevention services are available.

Mary's anxiety could be reduced by not engaging in activities or going out as often as before, but the nurse could support and empower her with the evidence related to the positive effects of exercise. Barker (2013) acknowledges that falls increase with age and can alter the dependence on carers and families. However, in the case of Mary, it needs to be identified that she is also a carer and therefore her support is reduced and her anxiety could be linked to concerns over her care responsibilities.

The NHS National Patient Safety Agency (2007) also stresses the need to recognise the impact of falls within a hospital setting. Hospital patients are at greater risk of falling than people in the community. Hospital patients may undergo surgery that affects their mobility or memory, and they may need sedation, pain relief, anaesthetic or other medication, which can increase the risk of falling.

- Older people are more vulnerable, and those who have fallen once are at a higher risk of falling again.
- Delirium increases the risk of falling and is particularly likely to affect patients on medical wards.

The Essence of Care provides indicators for best practice in relation to safety (Department of Health, 2010c).

People should be oriented to the care environment, taking into account their feelings, concerns, abilities, skills and cognitive level; the care environment is adapted (where possible) to help people feel safe and to reduce risk. Patient Safety First (2009) has developed a guide to reducing harm from falls in a hospital setting. Patient safety has to be balanced with independence, rehabilitation, privacy and dignity. *A patient who is not allowed to walk alone will quickly become a patient who is unable to walk alone.*

Conclusion

Looking after older people requires a great deal of skill. The complex needs of an older person require the nurses and the rest of the multidisciplinary team to be detectives to discover what is wrong and what are the most appropriate care interventions. This is an exciting area to work in and demands extensive nursing skills. This is what makes nursing the older person challenging, exciting, and ultimately very rewarding!

Activities: brief outline answers

Activity 5.2

Activities in a residential setting could include normal home-making tasks such as dusting, folding and putting clothes away; vacuuming (using a light-weight battery-operated vacuum if need be); cooking or preparing vegetables.

Men may prefer activities such as gardening and car maintenance (some homes have a car in the garden for men to 'tinker with'). Or a 'men's' club' could be organised where a rugby match could be watched with a few beers.

These are just examples and the request of the residents should be respected.

Activity 5.3

Some of the reasons might be:

infection; medication; pain; constipation; dehydration; change of situation; delirium; stress; anxiety; surgery; alcohol; poor vision and hearing; lack of sleep; lack of oxygen.

Activity 5.4

Routine observations will help identify if there is an infection.

Observe the patient: does he or she appear flushed and clammy, indicating a temperature? Or even cyanosed (blue tinge to the lips)? Confusion or disorientation could indicate hypoxia or lack of oxygen to the brain, which could signify a chest infection.

Can you hear the patient's breathing as you get nearer? Is the breathing noisy or laboured? Is the patient coughing? Are there a number of tissues scattered around? Is the patient producing any sputum? Again, a chest infection might be the cause. (If green sputum is being produced, send a sample to the laboratory for investigation.)

Are there any offensive odours that could indicate a urinary tract infection or infected diarrhoea?

Check for a rise in temperature, e.g. above 37.3°C. Even this low-grade temperature in an older person can indicate an infection.

If a routine specimen of urine indicates white blood cells or protein, a urinary tract infection might be suspected.

Activity 5.7

Use the SOLER techniques listed during your assessment to establish the best place to sit.

Identify a quiet place to conduct the interview.

Make sure Mr Jones has his glasses on and provide written information, in a larger font if necessary.

Examine his ears for the presence of wax and refer to the practice nurse for management of removal of wax.

Make sure the anaesthetist, surgeon and recovery team are aware of sensory deficits, and the need to speak clearly.

Useful websites

Action for Blind People: www.actionforblindpeople.org.uk

Practical help and support for blind and partially sighted people of all ages.

Age UK: http://www.ageuk.org.uk/health-wellbeing/doctors-hospitals/campaign-against-malnutrition-in-hospital

National Patient Safety Agency: http://www.nrls.npsa.nhs.uk/resources

NICE: http://www.nice.org.uk/nicemedia/pdf/CG021quickrefguide.pdf

Royal College of Nursing (2010) *Principles of Nursing Practice.* Available from: **http://www.rcn.org.uk/__data/assets/pdf_file/0011/349499/003863.pdf**

Royal College of Nursing, Nutrition Now: http://www.rcn.org.uk/newsevents/campaigns/nutritionnow/tools_and_resources/hydration

Royal National Institute of Blind People (RNIB): www.rnib.org.uk

Information, support and advice to people with sight loss.

SeeAbility: www.seeability.org

Supports adults who are visually impaired with multiple disabilities (learning, physical, or mental health).

Chapter 6
Psychosocial aspects of ageing

Lee-Ann Fenge

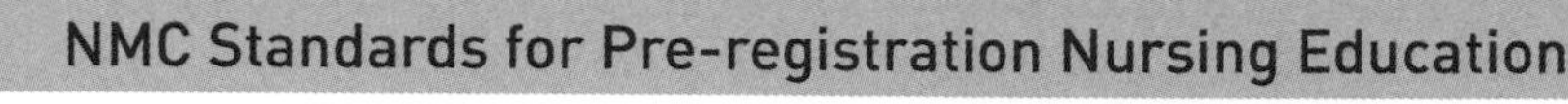

NMC Standards for Pre-registration Nursing Education

Domain 2: Communication and interpersonal skills

1. All nurses must build partnerships and therapeutic relationships through safe, effective and non-discriminatory communication. They must take account of individual differences, capabilities and needs.

Domain 3: Nursing practice and decision making

2. All nurses must possess a broad knowledge of the structure and functions of the human body, and other relevant knowledge from the life, behavioural and social sciences as applied to health, ill health, disability, ageing and death.
4. All nurses must ascertain and respond to the physical, social and psychological needs of people, groups and communities.

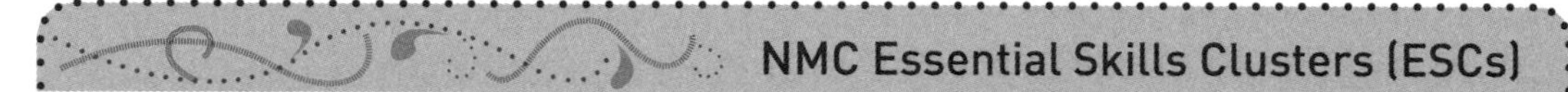

NMC Essential Skills Clusters (ESCs)

This chapter will support the following ESCs:

Cluster: Care, compassion and communication

2. People can trust the newly registered graduate nurse to engage in person centred care empowering people to make choices about how their needs are met when they are unable to meet them themselves.
3. People can trust the newly registered graduate nurse to respect them as individuals and strive to help them preserve their dignity at all times.
4. People can trust a newly qualified graduate nurse to engage with them and their family or carers within their cultural environments in an acceptant and anti-discriminatory manner free from harassment and exploitation.
5. People can trust the newly registered graduate nurse to engage with them in a warm, sensitive and compassionate way.

Chapter aims

By the end of this chapter, you will be able to:

- understand the impact of ageism and negative stereotypes on the way older people are treated;
- explain your understanding of the influence of psychosocial factors on ageing;
- discuss the impact of discrimination on the experience of older people;
- assess older people using a holistic biopsychosocial approach.

Introduction

Edna Walker died last week, aged 92, in her own home. Fiercely independent all her life, she had been a missionary in Africa and had never married. She coped independently without any outside support up until her sudden death from a heart attack. She was known to everyone in her village, and was a key member of the local church, holding the post of church warden until two years ago. She outlived her only sister, Ruby Evans, who was ten years younger; Ruby was a widow with no children, who never recovered from her husband's death when he was only 45 years old. She became depressed, and both her physical and mental state deteriorated as a result. Ruby needed support from carers and social services for the last 20 years of her life. Sisters can differ considerably in old age.

This chapter aims to help you explore what ageing means in our society and to use this understanding to inform and develop your nursing practice with older people. You will be introduced to both psychological and social factors which influence how ageing is experienced, and will develop an understanding of how such psychosocial factors influence how older people are seen and treated within society.

As a nursing student it is important you learn to recognise the complex relationships between medical, psychological and social aspects of individual experience. Birren (2007, p. 49) defines ageing as *interacting biological, psychological and social processes that start with birth and end with death.* You need to see past the biological changes in people to understand how these interact with the way society sees ageing and the impact this has on individual identity.

A recent King's Fund report suggests *patients need reliable holistic bio-psychosocial assessment* (Cornwell, 2012, p. 3). A focus on holistic assessment means recognising individual experience and countering the assumption that poor health and physical decline are an inevitable part of the ageing process, particularly when you are daily coming into contact with individuals in poor health within a nursing context. Many older people are enjoying an independent and fulfilling life in the community, and in self-reports, the majority of people over 80 say they are satisfied or very satisfied with their health (Oliver, in press).

> *The popular stereotype of old age as a time of universal and inevitable chronic health [problems] and impaired activity, is somewhat inaccurate. While the reported prevalence of a longstanding limiting illness*

> *increases with age, it is not a universal characteristic of later life. A little over half of men and women aged 85 and over living in the community report that they do not have a longstanding disability or illness that impairs their activity levels.*
> (Victor, 2005, p. 141)

If this is true, then it is important to understand why ageing is generally perceived so negatively in society, and the influence this has on the assumptions of nurses who work with older people. You therefore need to develop an understanding of both individual and societal influences on older people's experience, and an awareness of how ageism can impact negatively on the care that older people receive.

The use of terms such as 'elderly' may compound negative stereotypes about ageing, focusing on physical decline and loss and leading to assumptions that 'older people' are a homogeneous group with the same needs and aspirations (Tanner and Harris, 2008). Such an approach, alongside negative labels attached to ageing, contributes to older people being seen as a *social problem* (Thornton, 2002). In contrast, the use of terms such as 'elder' may dignify the maturity and wisdom which come with age (Hall and Scragg, 2012). It is important for nurses to separate the stereotypes and myths associated with old age from the real experiences of older people. As the Nursing and Midwifery Council suggests, *The essence of nursing care for older people is about getting to know and value people as individuals* (Nursing and Midwifery Council, 2009, p. 7).

Key elements of working with older people, therefore, concern:

- the need to combat ageism and develop person-centred approaches to working with older people;
- developing awareness of diversity on ageing experiences such as ethnicity, gender and sexuality;
- sensitivity to the impact of life transitions on older people.

Throughout this chapter you will be encouraged to reflect upon your own thoughts about ageing. However, to begin with it is useful to draw on older people's perceptions and experiences of their lives.

What is it like to be an 'older person'?

The first activity is in fact several: activities you can undertake to start to understand the experiences of being an older person.

Activity 6.1 *Reflection*

- On nursing experience placements, find older people who are willing to talk with you about their experiences. You should make it clear that you are interested in what they have to say as individuals, not just because of their age.
- Watch documentaries, films or TV programmes that depict the daily lives of older people.

- Talk informally with older relatives or friends.
- Read written accounts by older people, for example, autobiography, poetry.

As you undertake these activities think about the ways in which older people define themselves. What is it like to be old? What are the benefits as well as the difficulties of getting older? What aspirations or concerns do elders have about their future?

An outline answer is provided at the end of the chapter.

After undertaking Activity 6.1 you may have noticed that older people have many different perspectives and experiences of ageing, and may certainly have views which are different from those of younger people. However, as it is younger people who shape policy and the clinical environment, it is important for you to consider the stereotypes of old age and how these contradict the way older people think about ageing.

Thinking about ageing

There are different ways in which our society assesses a person's age:

- chronological age;
- social age;
- biological age;
- psychological age.

Every person has different ages by these measures, and they also offer us four ways of viewing old age, which is what we will do now.

Chronological age

We may define ourselves through chronological age, and this is the age on a patient's notes. But chronological age tells us very little about individual experience or levels of well-being. At what chronological age does 'old age' begin? As life expectancy increases, does the period we define as 'old age' also change? Chronological age denotes the number of years an individual has lived, but actually tells us very little about the individual's functional ability or individual circumstances. So, for example, a man of 95 years may be living independently and experiencing a better level of physical and social well-being than his nephew, who at 65 years has experienced a lifetime of chronic illness requiring support with daily living. However, chronological age can have an impact on the ways in which others perceive us, and it has been suggested that *ageism legitimates the use of chronological age to mark out classes of people who are systematically denied resources and opportunities that others enjoy* (Bytheway, 1995, p. 14). Chronological age also tells us which periods of history a patient has experienced, e.g. any patient born in the 1920s or 1930s has been affected by the Second World War.

Social age

We can also describe age in terms of key social aspects of ageing, such as entitlement to state pension, which change.

> *One of the ways our society defines age is through policy and entitlements. Social age also reflects the 'social construction of old age', which is the way in which meanings and interpretations and images that emerge from society affect the way we understand old age.*
> (Crawford and Walker, 2003)

This includes media representations of ageing as well as policy which creates or denies access to various resources, for example retirement pensions.

Historically, old age was defined by entitlement to an old age pension when a person retired from work at 60, later 65. Older workers' rights to remain in employment changed in the UK in 2011 when the default retirement age was introduced (Age Concern, 2011). You can now ask to continue working beyond the date when your employer wants you to retire, although the employer does not have to agree with this request. So people may remain economically productive past 65 years of age, and research suggests that the current economic recession is pushing some older people to remain in the workforce for longer (Munnell et al., 2009; Mountford, 2010). A recent report conducted by the insurance and pensions company Prudential (2011) suggests that 22 per cent of those delaying retirement are doing so because they cannot afford to retire. Therefore social definitions of 'old age' are fluid and change over time.

Biological age

We may also describe age in terms of our biological or physiological age, e.g. the loss of function in eyesight and hearing as we get older. Biological approaches to ageing understand age in terms of changes that occur as we grow older, and tend to adopt a negative view of ageing in terms of decline in function and ability across the lifecourse. However, biological changes do not occur in isolation, and the social and cultural context of the ageing body will have a big effect on how individuals make sense of themselves as they age. Access to a healthy diet, environmental pollution, smoking or drinking to excess can all influence how our bodies age biologically. It is therefore important to understand what it means to the individual to be experiencing an ageing body, and how this is influenced by wider social and economic experience.

Psychological age

Finally, psychological age is how people see themselves. For example, 'I may be 80 but I don't feel a day older than 35'. We all know people aged over 85 who 'help the old folk' at the over-60s club. How we perceive ourselves is influenced by the other three dimensions, and our sense of self and identity is co-produced to a certain extent by the images and feedback that we receive from society about our age, as well as the constraints of our own physical state. Older people bombarded by negative images of old age may see themselves in negative rather than positive ways.

Case study

Shirley Brown is 70 years old and lives with her mother, Ethel Brown, who is 88 years of age.

Shirley has suffered poor mobility for over 15 years due to arthritis. She has problems with daily living skills due to pain and limited movement in her hands, arms and legs, and rarely leaves the house. Her mother is very independent for her age and cares for her daughter, with limited support from social services. She tells everyone that she doesn't feel a day over 60! Ethel likes to do her own shopping, and still drives a car.

The Browns remind us that chronological age tells us little about someone's needs or abilities.

These different ways of conceptualising age demonstrate the range of factors which influence how old age is constructed and experienced. In the following exercise you will be encouraged to think about what 'old age' means to you.

Activity 6.2 *Reflection*

Think about the four different ways of viewing age. Reflect on how these relate to your own understanding of old age.

Think about the term 'old age' – what does it mean to you and what images do you associate with it? Make a list of these.

How many of these terms are positive and how many are negative? Why might this be?

At what age do you perceive 'old age' beginning?

What thoughts do you have about your own 'old age'? What are your aspirations and fears?

Think of the barriers to achieving these.

As this is a personal reflection, no outline answer is supplied.

This reflective activity enabled you to explore your own views of 'old age', as well as considering how stereotypical views of decline and loss might lead to barriers for older people in achieving their aspirations and life choices. The following section considers how ageism and discrimination can marginalise people within society.

Ageism and discrimination

As we saw in the previous section, the way we view ageing is influenced by biological, social and psychological factors. Old age is a social construct, and contemporary society tends to place a premium on youth whilst stereotypical views of old age are usually negative. It is important to understand how negative attitudes towards older people can lead to discrimination which undermines and disempowers them. Ageism may be reinforced by personal prejudice, cultural norms and values, and societal structures that reinforce social divisions within society.

Scenarios

Betty Hardwicke is 80 years of age and has recovered well in hospital following a fall and fractured neck of femur. She is now mobilising well, and is keen to get back home to her bungalow where she lives alone. However her son, who lives 100 miles away, has contacted the hospital to say that he doesn't think his mother should live alone at her age, and wants her discharged straight into residential care. Her son appears to have ageist views based on his mother's age.

Billy has suffered from depression all his life and has regularly attended a mental health day centre, which he enjoys. However, since he turned 65 years of age he no longer meets the centre's service criteria, and he will need to transfer to the day centre run for older people.

Power and discrimination go hand in hand, according to Thompson's personal, cultural and structural (PCS) model (Thompson, 1998). This model allows us to understand how older people can be disempowered within society by exploring three different levels at which power and discrimination operate: the personal, cultural and structural levels.

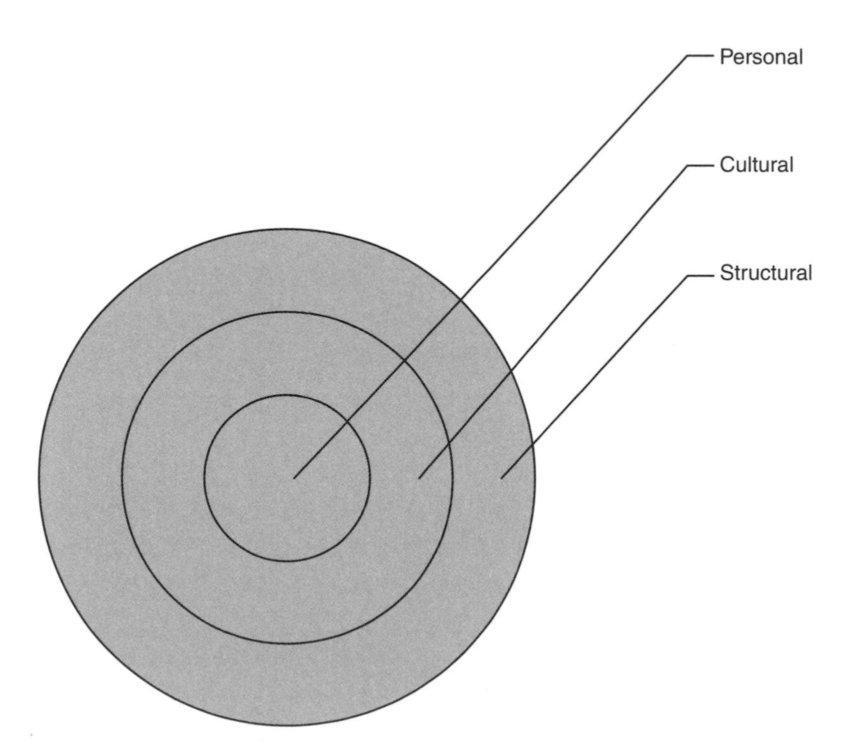

Figure 6.1: Thompson's (1998) personal, cultural and structural model

Personal level

Power operates at a personal or psychological level through a person's life experiences, resilience and ability to cope with changes and challenges in life. Those who have power over their own life are better placed to influence the circumstances they face. In nursing, this may involve enabling older individuals to develop confidence in their abilities and *to promote opportunities for well-being and psychological growth rather than helplessness and deterioration* (Nursing and Midwifery Council, 2009, p. 7).

Early life experience can influence later resilience to cope with transitions and change. For example, poverty earlier in the lifecourse has been linked to increased poverty in later life. Nearly 2.75 million older people occupy the bottom quintile of income distribution in the UK (Department for Work and Pensions, 2001) and the poorest pensioners are reliant upon the state for 90 per cent of their income, although a substantial number do not claim their full benefit entitlements (Victor, 2005). Better health and well-being are related to better economic circumstances in old age. This is true for various dimensions of health, including mental and physical health (Lum and Lightfoot, 2003).

When you undertake a holistic assessment, you should understand the individual within his or her own lifecourse, and how economic, social and cultural factors affect a person's own resilience and sense of control. High on the list of life experiences which damage personal power is any form of abuse or trauma.

Cultural level

The cultural context of ageing and old age concerns the level of shared meanings which carry with them sets of assumptions, stereotypes, language, imagery, and so on. Entrenched negative views of ageing and older people can be powerful forces which disempower older people within society, making them invisible and silent. Age discrimination is the most common form of discrimination in the UK, and *our view of older people focuses almost exclusively on biological decline* (Commission on Dignity in Care for Older People, 2012). How often do we hear that older people are a problem for health services, and an ageing population is a drain on resources that society cannot afford? Such negative cultural constructs of ageing often result in older people becoming powerless and dehumanised within care settings. Nurses need to challenge negative dehumanising assumptions about old age and recognise the uniqueness of each person in terms of his or her lifecourse journey (Todres et al., 2009).

Be on the lookout for an institutional culture in hospitals and other settings which reinforces negative views of older people, and may result in older people getting uneven access to the treatments and care that younger people experience. It is the nurse's job to challenge and change any such culture (see Figure 3.2 in Chapter 3).

Structural level

Age, like class, race, gender and sexuality, is a category which places people in a particular social position. Some positions have power, whilst others are often disempowered. Policy suggests a move away from ageist practice by providing services on the basis of need rather than age (Department of Health, 2001b, 2002). Successive governments have made older people's services a priority, most recently with the Equality Duty in the Equality Act (2010) dealing with age discrimination in health and social care coming into legal force. Policies and guidance to combat ageism, such as a National Service Framework for Older People, have been in existence for over a decade (Department of Health, 2001b). However, what is equally important is how such policy challenges and changes daily practice in healthcare. In order to combat ageism and challenge entrenched negative views about ageing we need to reflect on and question healthcare practice continually. Recent concerns about lack of dignity in care for older people highlight that older people continue to be subject to undignified and dehumanised care despite a raft of legislation to combat such practice.

Reflecting on the PCS model

The PCS model has been used to help nurses recognise and avoid discrimination. To explore and reflect on the PCS model, read the case study of Mr Grabski, which will allow you to recognise how it can guide your understanding and care of the older person from a psychosocial perspective.

Case study

Mr Grabski is an 87-year-old man who lives alone in a council house but has no surviving family. His son died at birth and a daughter was killed by meningitis in the 1960s, aged 18. Mr Grabski's wife died six years ago and he has been quite isolated since then. He lives on a state pension and has no savings. A female neighbour helps with shopping and errands, and she took on this role following his wife's death. He sought refuge in England in 1939 as a Polish airman and joined the Royal Air Force Volunteer Reserve – and has remained involved ever since. He has a basic state pension and also qualifies for pension credit as he has a low income.

Mr Grabski has been admitted to hospital after falling at home and fracturing his femur. He has repeatedly fallen at home previously while trying to get out of bed. He had not engaged with healthcare services since his wife's funeral, and is described as fiercely independent. He is described by the district nurse as 'difficult' to engage with. When she visited she found him living and sleeping in one room. She described him as having poor mobility – he used a broken broom handle to get around – reinforcing his social isolation (he used to attend the local Catholic church and Polish centre regularly). He had not bathed for some time as climbing the stairs and getting in and out of the bath were too much. He would wash in the kitchen sink. He often eats standing up in the kitchen because he struggles to carry his food, hold his stick and walk at the same time. He prefers to cook his own food and has refused meals on wheels in the past. He is distressed at being admitted to hospital and keeps saying that he wants to go home.

He was admitted to an orthopaedic ward, where he was described as 'difficult' and 'uncooperative', and the ward were keen that he be moved into a specialist bed under the care of the geriatrician. The view of the Sister on the orthopaedic ward was that he should be discharged into residential care.

Since being moved under the care of the geriatrician he has developed a positive relationship with the physiotherapist who is working with him to improve his mobility. He is keen to return home.

Activity 6.3 **Critical thinking**

Draw up a chart to analyse Mr Grabski's situation through Thompson's PCS model, to help you understand both power and discrimination issues in his case study.

An outline answer is provided at the end of the chapter.

You will have identified how personal, cultural and social factors influence older people's experiences and professional assumptions. The following section considers how some older people may experience multiple levels of discrimination because of ageism and diversity.

Diversity and ageing

Ageing experiences for minority groups

As earlier sections of this chapter have suggested, society is predominantly ageist and people are less valued, less visible and more powerless as they get older. Older people from ethnic minority cultures, those with disabilities or those who are lesbian, gay, bisexual or transgendered (LGBT) may experience multiple levels of discrimination. Such multiple levels of discrimination have been described as *double or triple jeopardy* (Cruickshank, 2003). It is therefore important to develop an understanding of how social divisions, such as those based on age, sexuality or ethnicity can make an individual visible or invisible within society. The way these different elements of identity intersect is described as *intersectionality* (Yuval-Davis, 2006), an approach which recognises the complexity of the interrelationships between biographical diversity and social context (Cronin and King, 2010). It can enable healthcare practitioners to develop an understanding of the diversity of social identities within the older LGBT population, and recognises diversity in the experiences of lesbian and gay culture (Hicks, 2008).

This chapter will use the example of sexuality to explore double jeopardy. Sexuality is often used to define people by terms such as heterosexual, straight, gay, lesbian, bisexual, transgendered, and such labels can act to marginalise individuals and groups.

It is difficult to know the precise number of older LGBT people in the UK population, although Price (2005) suggests an estimate of between 545,000 and 872,000 people over the age of 65. Heterosexism is a form of discrimination that favours heterosexuals over lesbians, gay men and bisexuals, and it can include the presumption that everyone is heterosexual.

Scenario

Imagine you are on the stroke ward where Bill, who is 78 years old, has been admitted. The stroke has left him unable to talk and with limited mobility. Every day he is visited by Jack, who you take to be his brother, as they are of a similar age. They appear very close, and Jack sits with him for hours, talking to him and

(continued)

continued ...

holding his hand. You often comment to Bill that he is lucky to have such a caring brother, but Bill never responds apart from shaking his head. After several weeks, you tell Jack that his brother is being moved to a rehabilitation ward, and at this point Jack says that Bill is not his brother but his partner of 40 years.

Heteronormative practice represents a viewpoint that expresses heterosexuality as a given instead of being one of many possibilities. For example, when working with older people we should not talk about their husband or wife but use the more neutral term partner.

Fear of heterosexism or homophobia may mean that older LGBT people often do not 'come out' to health providers and their needs are not recognised. Whatever the circumstances, it is important to accept that it is for individuals to choose how much information about themselves they share with others. It is not acceptable to seek information about someone's sexuality from a relative or friend.

Attitudes frequently lag behind the law, and the fear of prejudice and homophobia still lingers in people's minds. It is necessary to remember that the older generation of gay men grew up with homosexuality being illegal, and they may still live in fear. Although lesbianism has never been illegal, many older lesbians have had their children taken from them and/or endured physical, sexual and mental abuse because of their sexuality. Age Concern (2001) states that agencies which provide care for people often fail to take into account their sexuality. According to Age Concern's Opening Doors policy (2001), it is the organisation that needs to 'come out' as gay- or lesbian-friendly rather than depending upon clients to 'come out' in order to get their needs met. It is now against the law to discriminate on the basis of a person's sexual orientation, but well known that blatant discrimination is prevalent in care homes.

Bereavement may be particularly challenging for older people in same-sex relationships. Recent explorative research in Australia suggests that LGBT individuals face barriers in accessing appropriate end-of-life care due to discrimination and lack of knowledge about LGBT needs and experiences (Cartwright et al., 2012). Distress following bereavement may be increased if the nature of the relationship was hidden from family and friends (Rondahl et al., 2006), or not openly acknowledged by those around them. As a result, bereaved same-sex partners may experience the pain of 'silent mourning' or disenfranchised grief (Doka, 2002), and may be denied wider social and psychological bereavement support (Glacken and Higgins, 2008). It is therefore important that nurses are sensitive to the individual needs of every patient, particularly concerning relationships and loss. This means avoiding heterosexist assumptions about relationships, and ensuring that policies within practice do not discriminate against individuals or groups.

Activity 6.4 — *Leadership and management*

Age, like ethnicity, gender and sexuality, operates as a form of social division – it categorises people and plays a significant role in reinforcing how visible or invisible people are within wider society. Take some time to reflect upon the following issues and how they may influence nursing practice.

- What assumptions about ageing and sexuality may influence nursing practice?
- What impact might heterosexism have on an older lesbian or gay man?
- Consider the ways in which negative stereotypes and misconceptions about sexuality and ageing can be challenged and changed in nursing practice.
- How might you change attitudes of colleagues and build a service which promotes inclusion, self-expression and specific individual needs of older lesbians and gay men?
- What are the implications of the laws relating to homosexuality and discrimination on nursing practice?

An outline answer is provided at the end of the chapter.

This activity has enabled you to consider how certain groups of older people can experience multiple levels of discrimination, and has encouraged you to consider what implications this has on developing inclusive nursing practice. The following section will consider how nurses can support older people as they experience life transitions.

Supporting older people through life transitions

Older people often experience multiple transitions, such as those linked to loss of health, employment, status, home, relationships or loss through bereavement. Such losses may often go unrecognised despite leading to intense emotional responses. One model for understanding transitions is based on the control of the transition, and the expectation a person has about the nature of the transition. Four major types of transition are identified by Liddle et al. (2004):

1. predictable-voluntary (e.g. moving house);
2. predictable-involuntary (e.g. retirement);
3. unpredictable-voluntary (e.g. offer of parttime work);
4. unpredictable-involuntary (e.g. illness).

Looked at this way, we can see that unpredictable-involuntary transitions must be the most challenging for individuals to cope with when the transition is not only unexpected but is also out of the individual's control. Sudden illness or hospital admission falls into this category, which means that the individual may have difficulty coping with this sudden change, and may find hospital admission a threatening and frightening experience.

A key issue when working with older people in a nursing context is therefore to understand their experience of transition and how they are coping with it. This may include:

- deteriorating health;
- loss of independence, possibly increased dependence;
- feelings of loss of dignity, for instance, if support is needed for physical care;
- change of place (move into hospital ward).

Recent research suggests that older people in hospital settings not only experience 'care transitions' as they move across settings or services, but also experience transitions on a number of different levels, including physical, psychological and social changes (Ellins, 2012). To help you consider how coming into hospital or changing health status may affect an older patient, it is useful to consider the following model which describes seven stages of transition (Hopson and Adams, 1976).

1. immobilisation (a sense of being frozen, unable to act or understand);
2. minimisation (denial that change is important);
3. depression;
4. acceptance (realisation that there is no going back);
5. testing (trying out new behaviours to cope with the situation);
6. seeking meanings (reflecting on change);
7. internalisation (the new meanings discovered become part of behaviour and a new identity).

Of course not everyone will go through these stages, but it is useful to consider how you might develop your ability to support those who appear to be experiencing stress as a result of a life transition, and how they can be supported within a healthcare setting. The 'managing mechanisms' individuals use help them adapt to their changing situation. Such managing mechanisms can act as a 'protective force', which can prevent change and/or lessen the impact of it (Hill et al., 2009). People cope with transition in different ways. Our ability to cope is linked to psychological predispositions to stress and change; we also draw on a range of social, structural and economic resources. For example, an older women with a sensory impairment, living alone on a low income in poor-quality rented accommodation, would have increased vulnerability factors compared to a woman living as a couple in an owner-occupied house, with good family support and a private pension. The following activity enables you to consider how coming into a healthcare setting can trigger a range of transitions for older people.

Activity 6.5 *Critical thinking*

Consider the types of transitions that older patients might experience when they come into hospital or another healthcare setting.

- What personal factors might help patients cope with these transitions?
- What factors in the healthcare setting might support individuals to cope with transition?
- What factors in the healthcare setting might prevent the individual from coping with transitions?

An outline answer is provided at the end of the chapter.

The last activity encouraged you to consider how individuals experience transitions in different ways. Some older people may become very unsettled by life change, whereas others have more resilience to cope with change. Some individuals have been described as having increased 'hardiness' to manage life when under stress. A number of characteristics of hardiness have been described by Kobassa (1979):

- control: a feeling that one can control or influence one's life events;
- commitment: a feeling of deep involvement in and commitment to the activities of their life;
- challenge: experiencing life changes or obstacles as an exciting possibility for self-development.

It is believed that those with better 'hardiness' can better use coping strategies and manage stress, so are less affected by depression and poor health following stressful life events. This can also be linked to the notion of resilience. Resilience is a dynamic concept and may be seen as a process involving an interaction between vulnerability and protective processes that are internal and external to the individual, and which may act to modify the effects of adverse life events (Wagnild and Young, 1990). Resilience therefore can be seen as a kind of plasticity that influences our ability to recover and achieve psychosocial balance after adverse experiences (Richardson, 2002). As previous discussion of the PCS model suggests, resilience can be affected by earlier life experiences, and it is therefore important to understand older individuals within their life story or biographical context.

Case study

Gwen Forrest is 75 years old. She has been admitted to hospital after falling in the street where she fractured her wrist and sustained bruising to her face and arms. She has a large extended family, including six children, who between them visit her daily at home. She has many interests and hobbies, including singing in a local choir, and volunteering in the local charity shop once a week. She has previously suffered a heart attack and a mild stroke, and astounded the doctors by her positive outlook and quick rehabilitation back home following both these admissions. She is talkative and is described by the ward staff as having a sunny and positive disposition.

Activity 6.6 — *Critical thinking*

Consider how Gwen might cope with the transitions caused by her fall and injury, and her vulnerability or resilience to cope with this situation.

An outline answer is provided at the end of the chapter.

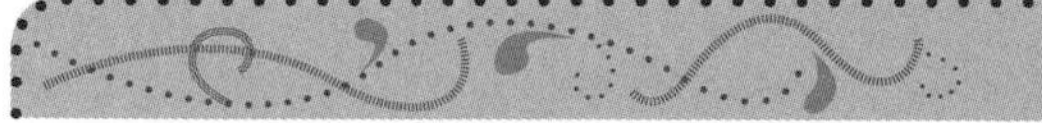

Chapter summary

This chapter has explored psychosocial influences on older people and how developing understanding of these can support you to work with older patients using a holistic biopsychosocial approach. It is important to understand how policy and practice are influenced by the way society sees ageing and this includes the ways in which older people may be discriminated against, not only on the basis of age, but also other elements of identity,

(continued)

continued ...

such as those related to gender, ethnicity, sexual orientation and disability. It is important to recognise that older people often experience many transitions as they get older, and illness and hospital admission may be a major cause of stress.

The key areas you need to consider in order to facilitate holistic biopsychosocial care are:

- the need to combat ageism and develop person-centred approaches;
- understanding of how biological, psychological and social factors work together to influence older people's lives and experiences;
- developing awareness and sensitivity of diversity on ageing experiences such as ethnicity, gender and sexuality;
- sensitivity of the impact of life transitions on older people and how health problems, and hospital admissions, may prove stressful for older people.

Activities: brief outline answers

Activity 6.1

It is interesting to reflect upon how older people define themselves, and you may find that, regardless of chronological age, people do not perceive themselves as 'old'. Some may perceive 'old age' as a period of opportunity whilst others may be concerned about growing older. Bytheway (1995) suggests that we need to understand individuals within the context of their whole lifecourse, rather than just using their age as a category. Research suggests that the ability to live an 'engaged life style' is an important component of successful ageing and well-being in later life (Betts Adams et al., 2011), although older people can be at risk of losing their social ties as they age (Heenan, 2010).

Activity 6.3

The PCS model allows us to consider a range on influences on Mr Grabski's experience. How might Mr Grabski's previous life experiences have contributed to his personal/psychological state? He has suffered many losses, including the loss of his homeland and family during the Second World War, the loss of both of his children, and more recently, the loss of his wife. This suggests that he may have some resilience to cope with life transitions. How empowered is he on a personal level? Living alone and being able to make decisions about how he wants to live his life, including taking risks, may be important for Mr Grabski. Making decisions about risk can make up a major part of older people's lives (Bornat and Bytheway, 2010). A willingness to take risks can be a crucial part of a person's sense of self-identity.

On a cultural level, negative dehumanising assumptions about old age may lead to assumptions that Mr Grabski should be more passive. He is described as 'difficult' by the district nurse and ward sister because he does not want to conform to their ideas about how he should live his life, and wishes to remain independent. How do cultural assumptions influence the care Mr Grabski might receive?

On a structural level, Mr Grabski is categorised by his old age, his Polish heritage and his male gender. For example, we may make assumptions about older men's ability to care for themselves, but expect older women to have little problem with the domestic aspects of their lives.

Activity 6.4

The Equality Act (2010) requires all public bodies and those performing public functions to:

- eliminate unlawful discrimination;
- advance equality of opportunity;
- foster good relations between groups.

It is important to consider how your work setting has responded to the equality duty in relation to older LGBT people. What training and other measures are in place in your work setting to promote understanding of the needs of older LGBT people, and to develop awareness of the discrimination they may face? Spend some time finding out about relevant policy and practice in your own work setting.

Activity 6.5

Coming into hospital can be a major disruption for older people as they enter an unfamiliar environment, and at the same time often feel vulnerable due to their health needs. They are removed from the routine and familiarity within their home environment to an often noisy and busy ward which can leave them bewildered. They may lose their independence quickly within an institutional environment in which they rely on others for care, and this loss of independence and confidence may compromise their ability to be discharged home in a timely manner. Think about how the ward environment or routines can undermine an older person's independence and confidence, and what can be done to alleviate this.

Activity 6.6

Gwen has experienced an unpredictable-involuntary transition following her fall and fracture. She appears to be coping well with this transition and currently appears positive in the hospital setting. She appears to have some resilience to cope with health problems, and to have recovered well from her previous heart attack and stroke. She has good social support, from both her family and social groups, and this adds to her resilience. She appears to have hardiness to cope with change due to the control she is able to exert and her engagement with her social world.

Useful website

Stonewall: www.stonewall.org.uk

National organisation that campaigns for legal equality and social justice for lesbians, gay men and bisexual people. Tel: 08000 50 20 20 (free from landlines).

Further reading

CSCI (2007) *Putting People First: Equality and diversity matters.* Available from: **www.cqc.org.uk**.

Department of Health (2007) *Reducing Health Inequalities for Lesbian, Gay, Bisexual and Trans People: Briefings for health and social care staff.* Available from: **www.dh.gov.uk**.

Ward, R, Rivers, I and Sullivan, M (2012) *Lesbian, Gay, Bisexual and Transgender Ageing: Biographical approaches for inclusive care and support.* London: Jessica Kingsley Publishers.

This chapter allows you to develop further knowledge about the needs of older LGBT people, and shows how your practice can be developed to be more inclusive of diversity within the ageing population.

Witten, TM and Eyler, AE (2012) *Gay, Lesbian, Bisexual and Transgender Aging.* Baltimore, MD: The Johns Hopkins University Press.

Although this is an American text, the chapter on intersex experiences provides insight into a little-researched area which requires particular sensitivity and understanding from healthcare practitioners.

Chapter 7
Mental health and emotional well-being in later life

Sue Barker

NMC Standards for Pre-registration Nursing Education

Domain 2: Communication and Interpersonal Skills

4. All nurses must recognise when people are anxious or in distress and respond effectively, using therapeutic principles, to promote their wellbeing, manage personal safety and resolve conflict. They must use effective communication strategies and negotiate techniques to achieve best outcomes, respecting the dignity and human rights of all concerned. They must know when to consult a third party and how to make referrals for advocacy, medication or arbitration.
6. All nurses must take every opportunity to encourage health-promoting behaviour through education, role modelling and effective communication.

Domain 3: Nursing practice and decision making

7. All nurses must be able to recognise and interpret signs of normal and deteriorating mental and physical health and respond promptly to maintain or improve the health and comfort of the service user, acting to keep them and others safe.

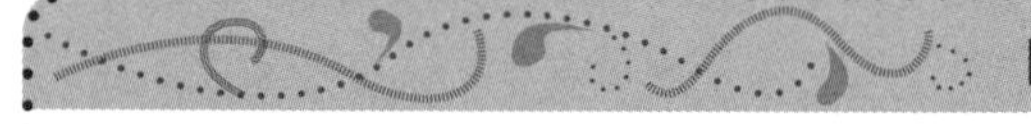

NMC Essential Skills Clusters (ESCs)

This chapter will support the following ESCs:

Cluster: Care, compassion and communication

2. People can trust the newly registered graduate nurse to engage in person centred care empowering people to make choices about how their needs are met when they are unable to meet them themselves.
3. People can trust the newly registered graduate nurse to respect them as individuals and strive to help them preserve their dignity at all times.
5. People can trust the newly registered graduate nurse to engage with them in a warm, sensitive and compassionate way.

Chapter aims

By the end of this chapter, you will be able to:

- understand the meaning of mental health and emotional well-being for older people;
- discuss the prevalence rates of mental health problems in older people;
- assess if an older person is struggling with mental health;
- understand the skills necessary to care for older people who have problems with their mental health or emotional well-being.

Introduction

There is a commonly held view in Western societies that older age brings depression and a low sense of well-being, but a report in *The Economist* in 2010 based on research in 2005 belies this.

> *Stiffening joints, weakening muscles, fading eyesight and the clouding of memory, coupled with the modern world's careless contempt for the old, seem a fearful prospect – better than death, perhaps, but not much. Yet mankind is wrong to dread ageing. Life is not a long slow decline from sunlit uplands towards the valley of death. It is, rather, a U-bend.*
> (*The Economist,* 16 December 2010)

The report identifies that the global average age for the lowest sense of well-being is 46, with the bottom of the U-bend being the 40s and early 50s. Most older people enjoy good mental health and sense of well-being (Lee, 2006).

Despite this, there are a significant number of older people who experience low mood and poor emotional well-being. The mental health and well-being of older people have been neglected in all areas – promotion, prevention and treatment (Lee, 2006) – and for many this causes suffering which is avoidable: there is much we can do to help. This chapter explores the prevalence of mental and emotional problems in older age and what you as a nurse can do to alleviate some of this suffering to support mental health and well-being. We will look at what has an impact on mental health and well-being in later life and how we might provide a humanised approach to nursing care. We look at the nurse's role in mental health and well-being assessment and screening. First, though, we need to establish what we mean by mental health and emotional well-being.

What is mental health and emotional well-being?

The terms 'mental health' and 'well-being' have been used interchangeably, according to the Mental Health Foundation (2012), and this may cause some confusion, particularly when assessing these as nurses. Take a few minutes to explore what mental health and well-being mean to you by completing Activity 7.1.

Activity 7.1 *Reflection*

What do you understand by 'mental health' and 'emotional well-being'? Make a few notes on what the terms mean to you. Either or both of them might mean:

- the absence of a mental disorder such as depression or anxiety;
- feeling happy;
- being content in yourself;
- enjoying being with friends and family;
- having sufficient money.

As this is a personal reflection, no outline answer is supplied.

If you think of mental health as the absence of a mental disorder or illness, you are in line with the biomedical approach to health (Wade and Halligan, 2004). This definition facilitates an objective assessment of mental health; the person could be assessed by a nurse or doctor using diagnostic criteria. In contrast, if you thought mental health was more about 'being content in yourself', this would require a more subjective assessment. Only the person could tell you he or she felt content, although you could look for signs of this in the person's behaviour. Your response could have been that all of the suggested states of being listed in the activity could usefully describe both mental health and emotional well-being. This would lead to an assessment using both objective and subjective measures. It would also suggest there is no difference between mental health and emotional well-being. It is important, though, that we consider the definitions available to us in the literature.

The Social Care Institute of Excellence (2005) identifies that well-being refers to our subjective assessment of how we feel about our life experiences. Given this definition you can see it would be difficult to determine the difference between well-being and emotional well-being. Our emotional state, according to their report, is usually accepted as fluctuating more frequently than our sense of well-being. They go on to imply that mental health and illness can be more objectively assessed. The definition of well-being that is accepted in this book is from the Department of Health (2007c, p. 99):

> *Well-being is the subjective state of being healthy, happy, contented, comfortable and satisfied with one's quality of life. It includes physical, material, social, emotional ('happiness'), and development and activity dimensions.*

As you can see, this encompasses all the states identified in Activity 7.1; it also includes mental and physical health. Mental health and emotional well-being can therefore be assumed to be part of overall well-being. The definition of emotional well-being accepted for this book is therefore: the subjective state of feeling healthy, happy, contented, comfortable and satisfied with one's quality of life.

A useful definition of mental health from the World Health Organization is:

> *Mental health is not just the absence of mental disorder. It is defined as a state of well-being in which every individual realizes his or her own potential, can cope with the normal stresses of life, can work productively and fruitfully, and is able to make a contribution to her or his community.* (World Health Organization, 2007b)

The World Health Organization definition focuses on coping, activities and development. Likewise, the Mental Health Foundation (2012) informs us that being mentally healthy does not just mean the absence of mental illness. It suggests that if you are mentally healthy you can make the most of your potential, cope with life and play a part in your family, work place and community and amongst friends. This is regardless of age, although your potential, coping strategies and the part you play with others are influenced by age. Imagine a two-year-old's coping strategies after being told she cannot have the toy she so desperately 'needs'.

Mental health is central to the totality of our health and influences the way we think, feel and interact with others. It affects our ability to communicate, to cope with change and manage challenges in our environment. McCulloch (2009) defines mental health as skills and strategies that enable us to function, which include thinking and feeling. Thinking allows individuals to plan, take actions, maintain relationships and value themselves, whereas feeling refers to the experience of satisfaction, happiness and contentment.

Older people identify that the following are important factors for maintaining their mental health:

- *Having a role and a purpose in life*
- *Having good social networks*
- *Enjoying an adequate income*
- *Living in a supportive neighbourhood.*

(Social Care Institute for Excellence, 2007)

Having a role and purpose in life links well with the concept of 'active ageing' or 'healthy ageing'. The World Health Organization (2002) describes 'active ageing' as the process of enhancing quality of life by facilitating security and involvement.

Older people believe that to age actively or to age healthily they need to:

- *Be able to adapt to continuous physical changes*
- *Engage in relationships*
- *Maintain independence and take risks*
- *Have enough money*
- *Fulfil desires and personal objectives*
- *Keep busy by taking part in meaningful activity.*

(Reed et al., 2003)

So there is a strong correlation between the factors that older people identify as important for maintaining their mental health and active ageing. Despite the recognition that older people have a sense of well-being, this is not the general perception of many nurses. As nurses, some of the older people we meet may not have a sense of well-being or healthy ageing, because of their poor health, although this should not be assumed. Therefore it is important that we identify how to help older people in our care to 'age actively'. The case study of Gladys Ravenhill should help you further explore mental health and emotional well-being.

Case study: Gladys Ravenhill

Mrs Gladys Ravenhill has lived alone for many years following the death of her husband fairly soon after he retired. She lives in a small terraced house and over the past few years the stairs have become too steep for her to climb safely. Her daughter and son-in-law have set up the front room, which had been kept only for special occasions, as a bedroom for her. She has two other rooms downstairs: a living room and a bathroom. A carer comes into her home every day to help her wash and dress and she receives a cooked meal each day through a home delivery service. Once a week she has an assisted bath. In her living room she has a large-screen television as her sight is quite poor. Her daughter, who works full time, visits her three times a week and her son visits on a Sunday morning. Her grandchildren visit intermittently. She has an emergency call service and is happy to use the telephone to keep in touch with her family. Occasionally she goes out on shopping trips in a wheelchair.

Gladys is seen regularly by the community nurse who monitors her various medications. Gladys does not seem to have problems remembering to take her tablets but she sometimes has problems at night when she says men come into her house underneath the locked door. Usually the men move things around in the living room and decorate for her. They do not come into her bedroom. A couple of times she has been concerned they may enter her bedroom and she has telephoned either her daughter or the police, all of whom reassure her there is nothing to worry about.

Activity 7.2 — *Critical thinking*

Reread the case study of Gladys Ravenhill.

- Do you think Gladys is mentally well?
- Do you think Gladys has a sense of well-being?
- Do you think Gladys has a good quality of life?

When trying to answer these questions, consider what you are basing your answers on.

An outline answer is provided at the end of the chapter.

Assessing Gladys, as to whether she is mentally healthy and emotionally well, requires complex skills. However, we do know that many older people who have had similar experiences to Gladys do have mental health and emotional well-being problems.

Prevalence rates of mental disorder in older people

As we have already identified, the majority of older people experience a sense of well-being and are actively ageing; the myth that it is normal to experience conditions such as depression and dementia is ill founded and unhelpful to us. There are, however, a significant number of people who do develop depression in later life (Table 7.1).

	Depression	Severe depression
People over 65	10–16%	2–4%
Over-65s living alone or in care homes with physical health problems	40%	

Table 7.1: Incidence of depression in later life

According to NHS statistics, the percentage of people experiencing a common mental disorder problem such as depression or depression with anxiety varies according to age and gender (National Health Service, 2007). People over 75 were the least likely to have a common mental disorder (6.3 per cent men and 12.2 per cent women) but these statistics were taken from people living in their own homes. For men the highest rate was the 35–44-year-olds (15 per cent) and for women, who generally had a higher incidence rate, the rate was highest at 45–54 (25.2 per cent) (National Health Service, 2007).

These are not the only figures that need to be considered when exploring the prevalence of mental health problems in older people; there are also a surprising number of older people with alcohol-related disorders, with the incidence increasing. The Institute of Alcohol Studies (2010) suggests that one in five older people have problems with drinking alcohol and the Mental Health Foundation (2012) estimates that 4–23 per cent of older adults being seen by medical staff have an alcohol problem. There are also 70,000 older people in the UK with a diagnosis of schizophrenia (Lee, 2007).

A mental health condition that has created a great deal of concern within health and social care recently is the expected exponential increase in dementia (Stephan and Brayne, 2008).

There continues to be some debate over whether dementia is a mental disorder or a physical disorder due to its organic nature but it is still classified under psychiatric disorders in the *Diagnostic Statistical Manual* version four (DSM-IV-TR) (American Psychiatric Association, 2011) and *International Classification of Diseases* version ten (ICD-10) (World Health Organization, 2010b). One in four patients in hospital have dementia (Alzheimer's Society, 2009) and the greatest risk factor for dementia is age (Table 7.2), so although there are about 16,000 people with dementia in the UK under the age of 65, this is a small minority of those with the disorder (Alzheimer's Society, 2012). Whatever their field of nursing, all students and nurses will have patients with dementia, not all of them elderly.

The case study of Gladys Ravenhill and the chapter so far have painted a mixed picture of the mental health and well-being of those in later life. Are older people enjoying later life with a

Age (years)	60–65	90 or over
Men	1.6%	Over 32%
Women	0.5%	Over 32%

Table 7.2: Age-related dementia diagnosis
(Source: the Mental Health Foundation website, 2012)

sense of well-being and high quality of life or is mental disorder rife? I am sure you will have noticed in previous chapters that people over the age of 65 are the least homogeneous group in our society and this is again the situation for mental well-being. Given the increasing number of people in this age group and the demographic information available we can assume that the incidence of people living into later life with health problems is going to increase along with those developing problems at this time. This does not mean that they will, or need to, experience a decrease in their mental health and/or sense of well-being.

Now you know about the prevalence of mental and emotional ill health, we need to consider what factors might influence these problems, so that we can start to address them.

What has an impact on mental health and well-being in later life?

Age Concern with the Mental Health Foundation (Lee, 2006) undertook a comprehensive inquiry into mental health and well-being in later life in the UK. This review found that there are a number of factors implicated in poor mental health and lack of well-being:

- discrimination – ageism;
- the ability to participate in meaningful activity;
- lack of relationships;
- poor physical health;
- poverty.

This list offers us the opposite to the factors identified earlier as necessary for positive ageing and health. Older people can experience psychological or emotional distress brought about by loneliness and isolation, loss of independence, retirement or unemployment, physical health problems and being widowed or divorced, all of which are risk factors for depression (Mental Health Foundation, 2012). Consider the scenario of Stanley Palmer and how the student nurse was able to make a difference.

Scenario

You are working, as a student nurse, in a stroke unit where you meet Stanley Palmer, an 84-year-old man who has had a left hemispheric stroke. He is having problems walking, swallowing and talking. When you first met Stanley he gave a wobbly smile to you, gained eye contact and was working hard to undertake the activities prescribed by the physiotherapist. After a couple of days he seemed to lack motivation for his activities and no longer attempted to smile or gain eye contact with anyone. You recognised these were signs that Stanley's mood may have become low. You asked the other members of staff if they had noticed the changes and you were told these are normal for someone with a left hemispheric stroke. Despite this you were concerned so you spent some time trying to engage Stanley in conversation. Through a few words and using his photographs brought by his family you found that his wife had been unable to visit him as they live in a small village with no public transport and she cannot drive. You also found out he enjoyed doing crossword puzzles. With this information you arranged for the hospital volunteer driver service to bring Stanley's wife in to visit him and bring in some crosswords for him. Within a few days Stanley was making improvements both in mood and mobility and was later discharged home with a holistic care package.

Whilst both men and women might have the same issues of maintaining emotional well-being, through relationships and meaningful activities, as Stanley in the scenario, the prevalence of these risk factors does have a gender bias. There are more women than men over 65 (about 100 men to 129 women), more men are married and fewer live alone or live in residential care (Williamson, 2011). Older men have fewer social relationships but women experience more physical health problems, financial constraints and social exclusion.

Social exclusion is not about poor relationships; it is about people being unable to access facilities. For example, if services are provided outside of walking distance, women are less likely to be able to get there as fewer older women than men drive. A more significant factor in the risk of mental distress, though, is social class. Those of lower social classes are more likely to have mental health problems and less likely to seek help early (Williamson, 2011).

Among the approaches to care for older people are the 'humanised approach' (Todres et al., 2009) and 'person-centred care' (Kitwood, 1997), which can help us as nurses help people regardless of gender or class. We have already looked at these approaches in Chapter 4 but in the next section we will explore these approaches in relation to mental health and emotional well-being.

Providing humanised person-centred care

In this book we advocate a humanised, person-centred approach to all nursing interactions; in this chapter this approach acknowledges the centrality of the person's experience. The individual is the expert and only that person can give an accurate evaluation of his or her well-being. Both Kitwood's early work on person-centred care (1997) and Todres et al.'s contemporary humanising framework (2009) recognise the individuality of each person on their unique journey through life and their need to be in relationships with others.

The majority of people with mental health problems cope on their own or with support from family and friends; they do not need the intervention of health services. As nurses using a humanised approach, we should encourage and support this. Self-help and peer support promote an active role for each person in their own recovery which is important for self-esteem. You can help promote the person's ability to help him- or herself by making life as normal as possible, with 'normality' identified by the person (rather than assumed by the nurse) (Lee, 2007).

Mental health services within the NHS have adopted a recovery approach to care which is supported by the UK government (Department of Health, 2001c, 2009c). A recovery approach is accepted as meaning helping the person in your care to [build] *a meaningful and satisfying life, as defined by the person themselves* where *hope is central to recovery* (Shepherd et al., 2008). Self-management and social inclusion, integral to recovery, are key factors in the establishment of agency (to be able to do something actively for one's self) and personal identity (Shepherd et al., 2008), which are important elements of both humanised and person-centred care. The recovery approach, person-centred care and humanised care all have a philosophy of care, placing the person in the centre.

The components of the recovery process are:

- finding and maintaining hope;
- re-establishing a positive identity;
- building a meaningful life;
- taking responsibility and control (Shepherd et al., 2008).

Shepherd et al. (2008) discuss the characteristics nurses need to facilitate recovery, which include good communication skills, positive regard, reciprocity and mutual regard and focus on the person's individual resources. This means you need to respect individuals and try to find out how they manage and cope with difficult situations and help them develop these abilities. Given the central importance of hope in the recovery process, you should try to inspire hope through your own life experiences and other people's. You can do this by thinking of a time you were in a similar situation or someone you knew was in a similar situation and explain how you or they overcame it. Consider how the nurse provided hope in the scenario of Anna Stone.

Scenario: Anna Stone

You have been asked to visit Anna, a 74-year-old woman who lives alone and has recently been discharged from hospital. Anna appeared frail, was moving slowly, looking at the ground and was rather dishevelled. You ask Anna whether she has any pain, to which she says no, and so you ask how things have been. Are things more difficult since returning home or are things easier since her hospital stay? Anna confides that actually it has been quite difficult returning home; she had enjoyed the company and conversations in hospital, although she had been irritated at the time. Anna was feeling lonely and useless. You explain to Anna that when you had an operation you had found it difficult to get back to normal and you felt quite low and tearful for almost two weeks afterwards. You tell her you slowly started going for a walk each day and each day the walk got longer and each time you went out you saw different people and chatted to them. You also tell how another woman you met had the same problems and she started attending a coffee morning at the local church which she found enjoyable and she went on to help by making coffee at the mother and toddler group. Anna thought both of the ideas sounded good and said she would try them.

The Mental Health Foundation (2012) offers ten ways to maintain mental health. You can apply them to yourself as a nurse and to the people you work with. They suggest you should:

1. Talk about your feelings.
2. Eat well.
3. Keep in touch with others.
4. Take a break from tasks.
5. Accept who you are.
6. Keep active.
7. Drink sensibly.
8. Ask for help when you need it.
9. Do something you are good at.
10. Care for others.

It is easy to see how you could facilitate some of these in your nursing through giving people the opportunity to talk about their feelings and the opportunity to ask you questions. You should ensure they are getting a good balanced diet and organise with them to take breaks if there are tasks they need to undertake. For individuals who are unwell it may take a lot of effort to get out of bed, washed and dressed in the morning so you could help them pace themselves and take breaks. It may be more difficult as a nurse to facilitate people accepting who they are, doing something they are good at and caring for others. These are, though, just as important for the person's mental health. If the older people you are working with have lots of energy they could do volunteer work such as gardening or shopping, but if they have limited energy they may be able to read to or listen to others. The most important way you can help others accept themselves is by you accepting them and treating them with respect.

Scenario: Jim Walkman

You are visiting Jim with the community nurse. Jim is 65 years old and has a learning disability. He lives independently but the community nurse is visiting him as he has recently been discharged from hospital and did not attend the GP follow-up appointment. When you arrive you find that Jim smells of alcohol. Jim agreed he had been eating chocolate bars and drinking alcohol.

Activity 7.3 — *Critical thinking*

Take a few minutes to consider the consequences in terms of physical and mental health of using food and alcohol as a coping strategy.

An outline answer is given at the end of the chapter.

When things are difficult people tend to use previously learnt coping strategies, regardless of their age. These are generally divided into adaptive and maladaptive strategies.

Adaptive coping strategies are those strategies that either remove the problem or allow us to reduce our distress despite the problem still being present. They can be further divided into emotion-focused and problem-focused strategies (Barker, 2007).

Emotion-focused strategies include going for a walk, relaxation techniques, singing, a warm bath; in essence, things that make you feel more comfortable and give you the opportunity to manage your emotions. Emotion-focused adaptive coping strategies can be helpful to the person when the problem cannot be resolved at the moment.

There are also numerous problem-focused coping strategies and they all consist of taking active steps to address the problem. If we return to the example in the scenario above, a problem-focused coping strategy for Jim would have been to seek support from his GP or the community nurse or for Jim to have asked for more information from the hospital staff before he left. As a nurse you will need to work with Jim to help him find adaptive coping strategies that he can put into place to help him manage or remove his discomfort. Working with Jim to establish his own coping strategies is person-centred and humanised and uses a recovery approach to his care.

Maladaptive coping strategies are those that have negative consequences for the person. An example of this is drinking alcohol to cope with psychological distress. A small amount may be beneficial, but exceeding the government daily recommendations can lead to significant health problems in the longer term and may cause dehydration, headache, nausea, vomiting, memory loss and disorientation in the short term. None of these are going to enhance a person's ability to manage discomfort.

Whilst it is easy to see how using adaptive problem-solving strategies is most beneficial, the advice from the Mental Health Foundation outlined earlier goes further than this. The ten strategies not only support a person coping with a difficult situation; they enhance a sense of well-being and may help prevent such problems arising in the future.

The Mental Health Foundation goes on to recommend self-help strategies for older people who are at risk of depression:

- *Take regular exercise;*
- *Plan for major life transitions such as retirement or moving home;*
- *Seek support from family and friends following the death of a long-term partner;*
- *Maintain interests, activities and social involvement, including learning.*

(Mental Health Foundation, 2012)

All of these strategies help us and the older people we work with, but many of our patients are already experiencing reduced well-being. So now we turn to ways in which we can recognise changes in well-being, and engage with people experiencing these changes.

Case study: Andrew Fowler

Andrew is 68 years old, a widower, and has recently retired from his job as a design engineer for a large pharmaceutical company. He developed paroxysmal atrial fibrillation when he was 64 years old and the practice nurse sees him every eight weeks to check his anticoagulation therapy through a fingertip blood test. His level has been stable for over a year. The practice nurse said he always smiles and makes the odd joke in his interaction with her. This morning the practice nurse asks Andrew's permission for you to undertake the blood test under her supervision. He consents to this but appears quite withdrawn. Whilst waiting for the small machine to give you the blood level and putting this result into the computer software you have the opportunity to discuss how things are going for him.

Activity 7.4 — *Critical thinking*

Take time to review the factors affecting mental health and well-being identified earlier in the chapter. What do you think the risk factors are for Andrew's mental and emotional well-being?

How might you start to assess Andrew's mental and emotional well-being?

An outline answer is given at the end of the chapter.

As you can see from the case study of Andrew Fowler, there are small indications that he may be experiencing a lack of mental health or well-being and we will need to undertake an assessment to determine how best to help him. The next section explores how to do this.

Mental health and well-being assessment and screening

Early detection is important for any health problem, and this is no less true of mental health problems. There are many assessment tools (see section below) available to nurses to explore the mental health and well-being of older people but the most important tool any nurse has is communication skills.

Using communication skills in mental health and well-being assessment

Nurses need to listen actively, showing respect, attention and compassion (Nursing and Midwifery Council, 2011). You do this through relationships with the people you are caring for. This special type of relationship is known as the therapeutic relationship. Rogers (1951) clearly outlines that a therapeutic engagement (developing a therapeutic relationship) involves:

- respecting the person;
- being genuine, trusting, sincere and honest;
- using good listening, attending and responding skills;
- being accepting (e.g. accepting another person's beliefs);
- having empathy (e.g. showing understanding of others' thoughts and feelings);
- being non-judgemental.

It is important to use this approach whilst conducting your usual comprehensive assessment. There are a number of approaches, such as the Single Assessment Process from the National Service Framework for Older People (Department of Health, 2007b), which is not considered in any depth here, but see useful websites at the end of the chapter.

Student nurses will have an identified assessment procedure and associated documentation for each placement. These will offer you the opportunity to explore how patients are feeling and if they are having problems with their thoughts. It is important to offer patients time to tell their 'story' in their own way as they may find it difficult due to the stigma associated with mental health problems. Consider how you might get Nancy to tell her story in the scenario.

Scenario: communication and engagement with Nancy

You are working in the outpatient department of a community hospital when you meet Nancy Swift, escorted by her daughter Susan. Nancy has just seen the surgeon for her six-week follow-up appointment; he is happy for her to be discharged as her wound has healed and she now only has a little tenderness in her abdomen. You are explaining about maintaining a high-fibre diet to Nancy, when her daughter says she is concerned about her mother as she has become progressively withdrawn since the operation.

There are a number of ways you may have chosen to respond to Nancy and her daughter Susan. You could have reassured Susan that it is normal to feel 'under the weather' after having an operation. You may even have thought this was an appropriate response to Nancy, and that may be so if you knew both of them well. It is important to obtain Nancy's version of what has been happening to her so you can ask her how she feels about it and if anything else is worrying her. This should be undertaken somewhere private and you should appear relaxed and interested, allowing her time to tell her story. You should show concern to both Nancy and Susan. Using active listening skills and respect should help Nancy to describe how she feels and why. Unless Susan spoke in confidence, you can say to Nancy that her daughter is worried about her; that might also encourage her to share her feelings.

If you are concerned about Nancy's mental health and well-being after hearing her story, you need to decide whether to advise Nancy to contact her GP or to contact her GP yourself, and there are many assessment tools that you could use to help in that decision. The next section explores some of the tools that may be available to you, but usually each clinical area has its preferred tools.

Assessment tools for mental health and well-being

There are a number of tools used to assess mental health and well-being in health services. As nurses we can seek guidance on which tools to use through frameworks such as the National Institute for Health and Clinical Excellence (NICE) guidelines for depression (NICE, 2007) or dementia (NICE, 2011). The National Service Framework for Older People (Department of

Health, 2007b) also offers valuable guidance on the need to assess and treat mental health problems. The assessment tools described below can be used within these frameworks.

Assessing depression

NICE (2007) states that nurses should take into consideration isolation, physical health and living conditions when assessing for depression in older people. It offers a couple of short questions nurses can use to gauge whether a person needs further assessment for depression:

- 'During the last month, have you often been bothered by feeling down, depressed or hopeless?'
- 'During the last month, have you often been bothered by having little interest or pleasure in doing things?'

If you are concerned about the person having mental or emotional problems, there are a number of psychometric tests to help guide your assessment of whether the person should be referred to specialist mental health services. There are three dominant depression scales that are used in health services: the Geriatric Depression Score (GDS: see below), the Hospital Anxiety and Depression Scale (HADS) and the Patient Health Questionnaire (PHQ-9). They have all been clinically validated and found to offer a good indication of distress. Your unit's own care pathways will determine the assessment tool you will use as a nurse.

The Geriatric Depression Score

The GDS has a number of versions which are labelled by the number of questions they hold. It is a scale used by all types of physical and mental health services with older people. GDS (15), (10) and (4) are all useful screening tools, but whilst GDS (4) is useful along with GDS (1), they have limited value as they do not assess the severity of the depression (Almeida and Almeida, 1999). They will, though, give you as a nurse some indication of whether further assessment is needed and can be used if you are short on time. If you only feel able to ask one question, then the one-question GDS can be useful. It is:

- Are you basically satisfied with your life?

You could expand this to a four-question GDS by adding:

- Have you dropped many of your interests or activities?
- Do you feel happy most of the time?
- Do you prefer to stay at home, rather than going out and doing new things?

(Almeida and Almeida, 1999)

GDS (10), (15) and (30) have even more questions and the 15-question version can be found at **http://www.stanford.edu/~yesavage/GDS.english.short.score.html**.

The Hospital Anxiety and Depression Scale

Another useful tool for assessing if the person may have mental or emotional problems is the HADS. This has been extensively used in physical care services, particularly acute hospitals. Copies of this can be found in many hospitals, and you can find it online at **http://www.surreyhealth.nhs.uk/dcp/Documents/D1.3d2.pdf**.

The Patient Health Questionnaire

The PHQ-9 is used in primary care settings to assess depression (**http://www.depression-primarycare.org/clinicians/toolkits/materials/forms/phq9**). It has nine questions that ask about mood, motivation, thoughts and behaviours. It asks whether these have been different from usual for two weeks. This scale is not specifically for older people but the signs and symptoms of depression are similar whatever the person's age.

Whilst these scales are helpful, particularly when providing a rationale for referral to specialist services, the key to recognising mental and emotional distress is your relationship with the person and giving the individual the opportunity to tell you his or her story in a safe environment.

Assessing dementia

Chapter 5 of *Dementia Care in Nursing* by Barker and Board (2012) offers a concise explanation of how to assess for dementia, but a brief overview is given here. Read the case study of Olga Robinson and think about whether you would consider her to be showing signs of dementia.

Case study: Olga Robinson

Mrs Olga Robinson is 75 years old and has been married to her husband for 50 years. Olga has found that since her early 50s her memory has deteriorated. She particularly struggles with finding proper nouns (names of things) when speaking, and more recently she has struggled with making decisions. When cooking she has missed elements of the process so she has served meals with various components missing, such as the vegetables or gravy.

Given Olga's history it would be difficult to make a decision on whether she has dementia, but there are a few indicators that she needs to be assessed for this as well as a number of other conditions. We will look at these after you have completed Activity 7.5.

Activity 7.5 — *Critical thinking*

Take a few minutes to consider what might be causing Olga's current difficulties, in addition to the possibility of dementia.

An outline answer is given at the end of the chapter.

Activity 7.5 shows that there could be health reasons other than dementia causing Olga's current difficulty. However, dementia could be a cause. The Department of Health clearly indicates that nurses need to be aware of the signs and symptoms of dementia so that diagnosis can be made as early as possible to improve the person's mental and emotional well-being and that of the carers. Principle 1 of the *Common Principles for Supporting People with Dementia* document (Department of Health, 2011b) outlines the early signs of dementia that healthcare workers such as nurses need to know. These are:

- loss or lapses of recent memory;
- mood changes or uncharacteristic behaviour;
- poor concentration;
- problems communicating;
- getting lost in familiar places;
- making mistakes in a previously learnt skill;
- problems telling the time or using money;
- changes in sleep patterns and appetite;
- personality changes;
- visuospatial perception issues.

As a nurse you will be involved in collecting assessments of Olga to assist in her diagnosis and treatment. Whilst the signs indicate she may have dementia, there are a number of other conditions that need to be ruled out, such as thyroid, renal and other mental health problems. There are a number of assessment tools that you could use to assess for dementia, but as with any other mental or emotional problems, it is your therapeutic relationship and communication skills that are crucial in ensuring a comprehensive assessment is made.

Psychometric assessment tools include: the Mini Mental State Examination (MMSE), the GP Cognitive Test (GPCog), the Six Item Cognitive Impairment Test (6-CIT), the Abbreviated Mental Test (AMT) and the Test Your Memory Test (TYMT) (see useful websites section at the end of the chapter for links). These can all be helpful in your assessment, or that of the doctor. Some of the most common questions in these tests involve assessing whether the person is oriented to time and place, with questions such as 'where are we now?' and 'what is the time/date?' They also involve short memory tests for recent and past information, such as giving the person a few words to remember, and then asking what the words were a few moments later. They also involve assessment of concentration, attention and visuospatial abilities.

Whilst it is unlikely that you, as a nurse, will be making the final decision on a diagnosis of the person you will be involved in gathering information and supporting the person through this process. It is also most likely to be you who will provide any care they may need.

This section has explored the screening of mental health and emotional well-being and the next section will go on to consider what nursing care may be required and how it should be provided.

Nursing care

In 2005 the Joseph Rowntree Foundation funded an inquiry called That Little Bit of Help to find out how older people's well-being could best be supported (Raynes et al., 2006). This inquiry gathered information from not only academics, practitioners and commentators, but also from older people; in fact it gathered more comments from older people than from any other group. The inquiry showed that older people are not a problem that needs resolving, but a major care provider. This research, along with the follow-up schemes such as LinkAge Plus and Partnership for Older People Project (POPP), has added to our understanding that even minimal early intervention can enhance quality of life and well-being in older people; for example, small tasks such as help with shopping have a big impact (Knapp, 2010). There are many small actions that can be undertaken to improve well-being within all care settings, whether that is the person's own home, warden-assisted accommodation, residential homes, nursing homes or hospitals. You as the nurse providing care should therefore be aware of these opportunities to make a difference. When we are involved in any interaction with an older person we need to:

- Listen to what they are saying.
- Recognise their capacity to help themselves.
- Provide opportunities for meaningful activity and social engagement.
- Develop peer support.
- Develop information and advocacy services.
- Integrate formal and informal services.
- Develop our understanding of recovery, offering hope to the person and carer (Lee, 2007).

In the following discussion we will look at how you can provide nursing care in each of these areas; you also need to develop health promotion opportunities and ensure supportive settings for care for the older person to improve well-being.

Listening to what the person is saying

Whatever the care setting, it is crucial that the older person and family or carer are central to decision making. We have already explored this earlier in the chapter but it is worth highlighting again here – whenever you are providing nursing care with the older person, utilise your listening skills to explore opportunities to enhance the person's well-being and mental health. This was considered in the scenario related to Nancy Swift. With Nancy you saw that behaving respectfully and with concern allowed her to share her story but it is also important to show that you have listened by acting on the information you are given. If Nancy says she finds watching television causes her to feel dizzy and confused, do not ask her to wait in a room with a television on.

Recognise a person's capacity to help him- or herself

As identified earlier, there are many ways in which older people can help themselves to maintain their own mental and emotional well-being (see list from the Mental Health Foundation, 2012), so as a nurse you should explore their capacity to undertake these before planning other nursing interventions. You could assess how they can undertake regular exercise; there are a wide variety of ways this can be achieved. Walking is an excellent activity but for people who are unable to mobilise easily there are armchair exercises.

Provide opportunities for meaningful activity/social engagement

One key initiative identified by the schemes mentioned at the start of this section is befriending services (Raynes et al., 2006; Knapp, 2010). These services offer the opportunity for increased well-being and health for both the befriender and the befriended. This aligns with the recommendations by the Mental Health Foundation, Kitwood's (1997) person-centred care and Todres et al.'s (2009) humanised care (seen earlier in this chapter), all of which recognise the importance of relationships with other people for good mental health and well-being. It is therefore important that we, as nurses, help older people to meet and chat to each other. We can easily do this by involving the families and carers, with the person's permission, in developing any planned care.

You need to delve gently into a person's life and character to assess what is a meaningful activity for them: never make assumptions based on generalities. Each person is unique.

Develop peer support

Older people, as we have seen, are actually the biggest group of care givers to older people (Raynes et al., 2006). Older people themselves provide valuable services, often as volunteers, or informally as grandparents or carers, where they can be recognised for their warmth and wisdom. Sometimes the roles of carer and the cared-for become mixed.

Case study: Vera Jones

Vera is 83 years old and a widow; she has been attending the same church for over 50 years. When she was younger she used to enjoy leading the children's activities. Vera always sits in the same pew, always smiles at people as they enter and leave church and engages with the prayers and hymns with enthusiasm. Vera appears gentle and friendly.

Sue, a woman of 65, another church-goer, was having a difficult week; work was getting on top of her and she was worried about her children despite their leading independent lives. As she entered church Vera smiled at her and Sue felt the warmth of the smile and was comfortable in joining Vera in her usual pew. Vera noticed Sue was a little distressed, and smiled and touched her hand. Sue became tearful and Vera sat and listened to Sue's worries and concerns, and gave her a warm smile and a hug. When Sue left church that day she felt cared about and listened to. When most of the people had left the church Vera's carer came to collect her. She was unable to find her way home because of her dementia, but she continued to be encouraged by others and able to encourage others.

The case study of Vera Jones shows that all of us need care, at times, and to achieve mental health and emotional well-being we need in turn to care for others, regardless of our age. Vera was able, despite her dementia, to offer peer support to another woman considered by our society to be an older person. There are many more examples of older people offering support and care to other older people. It is therefore not difficult to see that as nurses we need to engage with older people actively to identify the knowledge and skills they have and wish to share. We need to use our imagination to facilitate peer support, which could also be a meaningful activity for the older person. As identified throughout this chapter, everyone gains satisfaction from being of use to others, and older people are no exception.

Develop information and advocacy

All of the sections dealing with care are interrelated and have a common theme. Probably the best people to offer advocacy and information to older people is older people themselves, and we should facilitate this when we can by supporting the development of schemes such as LinkAge and POPP, mentioned earlier. We may also be able to develop such links through coffee mornings and support groups, depending on where we work. In situations where older people are unavailable to offer information and advocacy, we need to provide it ourselves. To do this we need to ensure the information, whether verbal or written, or via electronic media, offers a clear understanding and is appropriate for the audience. As people age their perceptual abilities such as sight and hearing decrease so when giving information you must ensure the person can access it. Information should be relevant, accessible, timely and coordinated (Lee, 2007). Remember, most older people do not have internet access and many do not use mobile or smart phones.

As nurses we are compelled by our professional body to advocate for those in our care (Nursing and Midwifery Council, 2011). Advocacy is about giving people the right to make their own decisions (Lee, 2007). We can do this informally as well as formally; we can formally set time aside when older people can approach us or, in individual circumstances, we can approach them. We should also be an advocate in all areas of our work, ensuring the older person's voice is heard, such as in case reviews or in service planning meetings. We can also challenge others who have negative attitudes towards older people. Let us not pretend this does not occur in hospitals every day.

Scenario: Amelia Twinning

Amelia gets very tired if she needs to walk any distance so you have taken her in a wheelchair to the X-ray department. When you arrive, the receptionist ask you, 'What is her name?' and 'Do you have her notes?' and says, 'Take her over there to wait'. The receptionist does not speak to Amelia at all. How do you think this might affect Amelia's emotional well-being?

The receptionist in the scenario above could be considered efficient, quickly processing people through the unit, but you know that Amelia might have experienced reduced self-esteem and self-worth in this situation. If you believed that Amelia's mental and emotional well-being might be adversely affected by this interaction you should have intervened. You could have done this in a non-confrontational way; each time you were asked a question, you could in turn ask Amelia and seek her consent. You could also have chosen to say to the receptionist that you are only there to assist Amelia and she should ask Amelia for any information she needed. Information giving and advocacy are important parts of our role as nurses. They can be formal, and address a large group, or they can be informal and provided in an individual, personalised way.

Integrate formal and informal services

It is important that nursing care for older people is provided using a collaborative approach; indeed, our professional body states we need to do this (Nursing and Midwifery Council, 2010), particularly between primary care, social care and mental health services. This is especially important if the person has mental or emotional problems (Lee, 2007). This should ensure timely responses to need and reduce the stress put on the older person. Collaborative care and interprofessional working are discussed in more detail in Chapter 10. It is important that nurses work collaboratively with the person, family and carers, and with other professionals such as social workers, doctors and occupational therapists.

A collaborative approach across formal and informal services should facilitate early detection of mental and emotional problems, which can lead to more choices and reduce distress.

Offer hope to the person and carer

Offering hope to the older person and family is probably the most important thing we can do; a lack of hope is linked to depression and suicide (Norman and Ryrie, 2009). The provision of hope is central to the recovery approach in mental health services and is implicit within person-centred and humanised care. We provide hope by being optimistic for the person and seeking ways to solve problems and provide comfort. All the areas so far considered under the heading of care can provide people with a sense of hope: being listened to, recognising there is something they can do for themselves, having meaningful activities, having relationships, being cared about and being able to care for others, being advocated for and being given accurate information on diagnosis and treatment.

Develop health promotion opportunities

Nurses can have ongoing care relationships with older people for whom the usual health promotion issues, such as nutrition, exercise, smoking and substance abuse (including alcohol) cessation, are extremely important to enhance well-being. As identified earlier in the chapter, physical health problems, isolation and poverty are key issues in maintaining mental and emotional health. Therefore use any opportunity that you can to provide health promotion support and advice.

Ensure supportive settings for care

Nurses care for older people in a variety of settings, in each of which may be different sets of issues that may affect well-being. In the hospital environment the older person's self-efficacy may be reduced by mobility, lighting, noise and high beds, all of which reduce self-esteem. With a little thought you can deal with these. Nursing staff and healthcare assistants can reduce the noise of closing doors, clanging bins and loud conversation. For the older person who is a little disoriented due to cognitive impairment, physical or mental health problems, try using clocks, calendars and pictorial guides (Lee, 2007). Listen to patients: use your imagination; help adjust their experiences and improve their quality of life. We know we should behave towards others in the way we would like to be treated, but as nurses we need to go further than this; we need to identify how people as individuals like to be treated. Older people are the least homogeneous group in our society, and their hopes, expectations and needs are very different from each other, so we should not expect them all to be the same as our own or each other's.

Transitions between care environments can be traumatic for the older person, whether that is between home and residential care, or residential care and hospital care, or the other way around. This can lead to feelings of loss of belongings and relationships, reduced quality of life, lack of sense of identity and reduced ability to engage in meaningful activity (Lee, 2007). We need to acknowledge this and be prepared to support the older person through this difficult time, utilising both problem-solving and emotional coping approaches, identified earlier in the chapter.

In this section we have explored Lee's (2007) important areas of interaction to develop mental and emotional well-being and have established how we, as nurses, can make a difference in these areas.

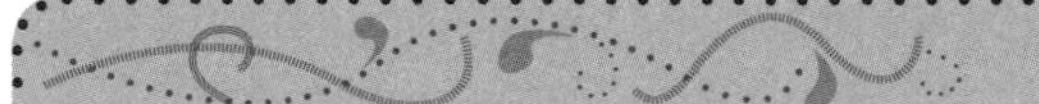

Chapter summary

Although people often think that older age equates with a low sense of well-being, this is not the case for most older people. This myth, though, has led to a limited focus on helping older people who do experience reduced mental health and emotional well-being. There is much that can be done to help older people in this situation. Mental health and emotional well-being have been identified as being mostly subjective, but there are some validated assessment tools such as the GDS and the MMSE to guide the nurse's assessment of mental health. The main tool, though, available to nurses in the assessment of mental health and emotional well-being is their therapeutic relationship and communication skills.

How you, as a nurse, can achieve emotional well-being in older people involves listening to the person, being imaginative, understanding that even small actions can make a difference and sharing your hope.

Activities: brief outline answers

Activity 7.2

Do you think Gladys is mentally well? It is very difficult to assess whether Gladys has mental health problems from this case study; she may be experiencing hallucinations and delusions or it may be that she hears noises in the night and interprets them as people in her house. If she then finds that house looks slightly different, either because the carer has tidied up before leaving or because of minor cognitive impairment, it adds weight to her interpretation that there were people in her house.

Do you think Gladys has a sense of well-being? This is again difficult to assess without asking her; as defined earlier in the chapter, well-being is a subjective experience so it would be unwise to assume that if a person has health problems that interfere with the activities of daily living she has a reduced sense of well-being.

Do you think Gladys has a good quality of life? Again, this is difficult to assess with the information provided here. Despite Gladys not having the things in her life that you as a nurse might desire for quality of life, that does not mean that she desires the same things.

Activity 7.3

The use of food and alcohol as coping strategies for stress and anxiety is quite common in our culture and may be useful in the short term, but in the long term can present health problems.

Chocolate is high in fat, over-consumption of which can lead to obesity, a big contemporary health concern; one in four adults and over one in ten children are obese (Department of Health, 2012). Obesity can lead to type 2 diabetes, some cancers, heart and liver disease (Department of Health, 2012).

Alcohol can give a feeling of reduced stress and anxiety but can lead to *damage of the brain and nervous system, affect immune system, harm bones, skin and muscles, cause fertility problems and impair foetal development* (Scotland.gov., 2010, p. 1).

Activity 7.4

The factors that could indicate that Andrew may be at risk of reduced mental and emotional well-being are:

- being widowed;
- recent retirement;
- an income that has probably reduced;
- ongoing health problems.

As part of your assessment of Andrew you could ask him how he is feeling and whether there have been any recent changes. You could also ask him if he is happy with life at the moment. The important thing is to allow Andrew time to share his thoughts and feelings in his own way.

Activity 7.5

There are a number of possibilities for the cause of Olga's current problems and finding out over what period of time they have developed is crucial in determining the cause. If the problem has occurred quite quickly it may be due to an infection or stress. If the problem has developed more insidiously it may be due to hormonal changes or dementia. It is therefore important to undertake a comprehensive assessment of her health.

Useful websites

http://www.depression-primarycare.org/clinicians/toolkits/materials/forms/phq9

This website explains the PHQ-9 assessment tool for assisting practitioners in primary care to identify depression. It has two components: assessing symptoms and functional impairment and also severity. The tool can be used to monitor response to treatment as well.

http://www.patient.co.uk/health/Memory-Loss-and-Dementia/professionalpatient.co.uk

This website offers access to a variety of assessment tools to assess dementia as well as links to other related information on dementia.

http://www.surreyhealth.nhs.uk/dcp/Documents/D1.3d2.pdf

This pdf is a copy of the HADS that is used widely throughout hospitals in the UK, but again it is only an indicator that people need further assessment. This is a useful tool, not specifically for older people but for all adults.

http://webarchive.nationalarchives.gov.uk/+/www.dh.gov.uk/en/SocialCare/Chargingandassessment/SingleAssessmentProcess/DH_079509

The Single Assessment Process was introduced by the government in 2001 and details of it can be found in the national government archives. It is a process recommended by the National Service Framework for Older People (Department of Health, 2007b).

Further reading

Barker, S and Board, M (2012) *Dementia Care in Nursing.* London: Sage/Learning Matters.

This book explores all areas of dementia nursing, including assessment, differential diagnosis and care. It is written with clarity and, as with this book, is linked to the nursing competencies set by the Nursing Midwifery Council in 2010.

Pratchett, T (2011) Diagnosing Clapham Junction syndrome. In Grant, A, Biley, F and Walker, H (eds) *Our Encounters with Madness.* Ross-onWye: PCCS Books, pp. 160–164.

Sir Terry Pratchett is a famous author who has dementia. This chapter offers an insight into his response to having this disease. He is very cross about it but, as with his famous 'Discworld' novels, this piece is written in his everyday language and prompts laughter and tears. It also offers the human experience that has not been sanitised by academics.

Williamson, T (2011) Grouchy old men? Promoting older men's mental health and emotional wellbeing. *Working with Older People,* 15 (4): 164–176.

This journal article brings together policy, research and practical service improvement initiatives. It describes a project undertaken over two years but also offers a good review of the relevant literature.

Chapter 8
Ageing in a multicultural society

Janet Scammell

NMC Standards for Pre-registration Nursing Education

This chapter will address the following competencies:

Domain 1: Professional values

2. All nurses must practise in a holistic, non-judgmental, caring and sensitive manner that avoids assumptions, supports social inclusion; recognises and respects individual choice; and acknowledges diversity. Where necessary, they must challenge inequality, discrimination and exclusion from access to care.

Domain 2: Communication and interpersonal skills

1. All nurses must build partnerships and therapeutic relationships through safe, effective and non-discriminatory communication. They must take account of individual differences, capabilities and needs.
2. All nurses must use a range of communication skills and technologies to support person-centred care and enhance quality and safety. They must ensure people receive all the information they need in a language and manner that allows them to make informed choices and share decision-making. They must recognise when language interpretation or other communication support is needed and know how to obtain it.

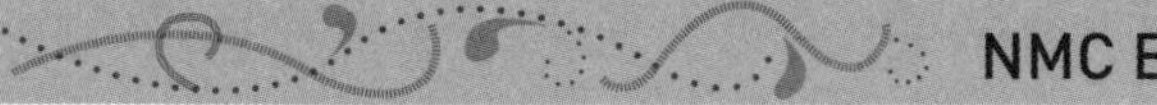

NMC Essential Skills Clusters (ESCs)

This chapter will address the following ESCs:

Cluster: Care, compassion and communication

4. People can trust a newly qualified graduate nurse to engage with them and their family or carers within their cultural environments in an acceptant and anti-discriminatory manner free from harassment and exploitation.

By the first progression point

1. Demonstrates an understanding of how culture, religion, spiritual beliefs, gender and sexuality can impact on illness and disability.

(continued)

continued ...

By the point of entry to the register

5. Is acceptant of differing cultural traditions, beliefs, UK legal frameworks and professional ethics when planning care with people and their families and carers.
6. Acts autonomously and proactively in promoting care environments that are culturally sensitive and free from discrimination, harassment and exploitation.

Chapter aims

After reading this chapter, you will be able to:

- understand the demographics associated with age and ethnicity in the UK and its relevance to care provision;
- describe the common terms used in relation to cultural diversity and care;
- explain the reasons for health inequalities related to ethnicity;
- apply the humanising values framework to care of clients from diverse cultural backgrounds.

Introduction

> *There is little difference in people, but that little difference makes a big difference. The little difference is attitude. The big difference is whether it is positive or negative.*
> (W. Clement Stone, businessman, author, philanthropist)

The UK is a multicultural society. Recent population census data indicate that ethnic diversity in older age groups has increased significantly (see Figure 8.1 on page 146) over the last century (Office for National Statistics, 2013). All nurses, regardless of their own cultural and ethnic identity, must be knowledgeable and responsive to the needs of older people from differing backgrounds. It is vital that as nurses we develop appropriate knowledge, skills and attitudes to work with and care for everyone, including those we perceive to be 'different' from ourselves. Most of us would claim we do not discriminate on the basis of what people look like or believe, or how they speak, and that we always treat everyone equally, but the evidence is that some of us do. Whilst overt discrimination has become rare in recent years, negative attitudes are not; these can lead to a more insidious, if unwitting, form of discrimination that can contribute to poorer health and well-being in certain groups in society. This chapter will consider some of the knowledge and skills that the nurse requires to provide effective, compassionate and culturally acceptable care for older people.

The chapter begins by outlining the structure of the UK population, focusing on age and ethnicity. Common terms are defined and explained as part of the context for exploring the needs of differing ethnic groups. Health inequalities between different ethnic groups are described and some explanations offered. Perceptions of ageing across different cultures are then compared, including attitudes to ageing and care in older age. Some inequalities are associated with misplaced assumptions about people from ethnic groups that differ from our own. It will be suggested that focusing on the central tenets of what it means to be human rather than on perceived group differences may enable nurses to respond in a more inclusive, caring and compassionate manner to all patients. This is explored through the application of the humanising values framework.

The UK: an ageing and ethnically diverse society

Over the last century the structure of the UK population has changed significantly. The Office of National Statistics (ONS) surveys the size and composition of the total population every decade, the last census being in 2011. The composition of the population as determined at the census time is determined by three interrelated factors, namely patterns of births, deaths and migration that have taken place in the previous ten years.

Older age population profile

Compared to the 2001 data, the structure of the population of England and Wales in 2011 remains broadly similar, with the percentage of the population aged 65 and over increasing by 0.5 to 16 per cent of the total population. Although the very old (aged 90 and over) form under 1 per cent of the population, their numbers increased by 26 per cent between 2002 and 2011. However, over the last century the UK population structure has changed significantly due to the impact of the declining birth and mortality rates recorded across the 100-year period. The proportion of older people aged 65 and over has more than trebled from 5 per cent in 1911 to 16 per cent in 2011 (Figure 8.1). The trend of increasing numbers in the older age groups has clear implications for the provision of healthcare.

Ethnic population profile

The British Isles has become the home for migrants from other lands throughout its history. The 2011 census reported that, whilst the majority of the UK population belongs to the white British ethnic group, 12 per cent (2 million) of households with at least two people had partners or household members of different ethnic groups. Looking at the data for England and Wales, 86 per cent of the population stated their ethnicity as white. The majority of this group was white British, with 5 per cent comprising white minority ethnic groups. Minority ethnic groups are all groups excluding white British and comprise 19 per cent of the UK population. The main ethnic groups apart from white British and white minority ethnic groups (for example, Irish, Gypsy and Irish Travellers) are mixed ethnic group, Asian/Asian British, black/African/African Caribbean/black British and other ethnic group (for example, Chinese) (Figure 8.2).

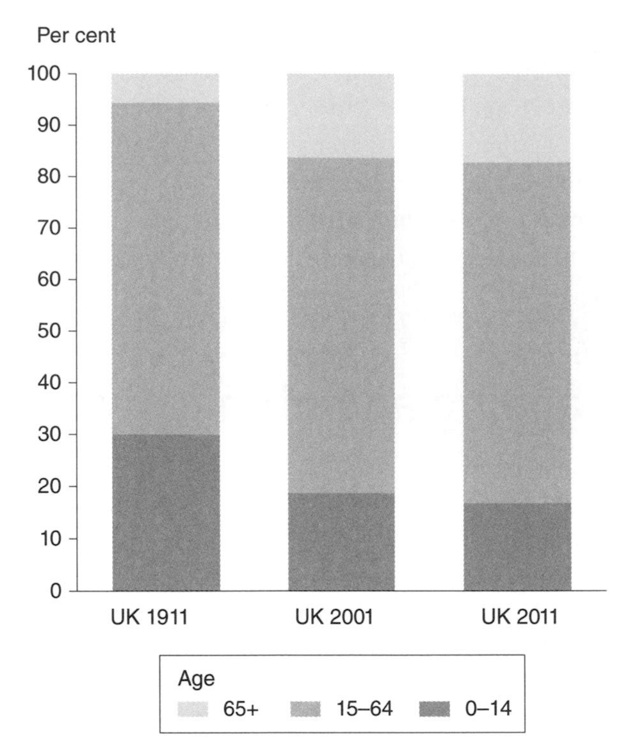

Figure 8.1: UK population by broad age group: 1911, 2001 and 2011

(Source: Office for National Statistics, 2012a, with permission)

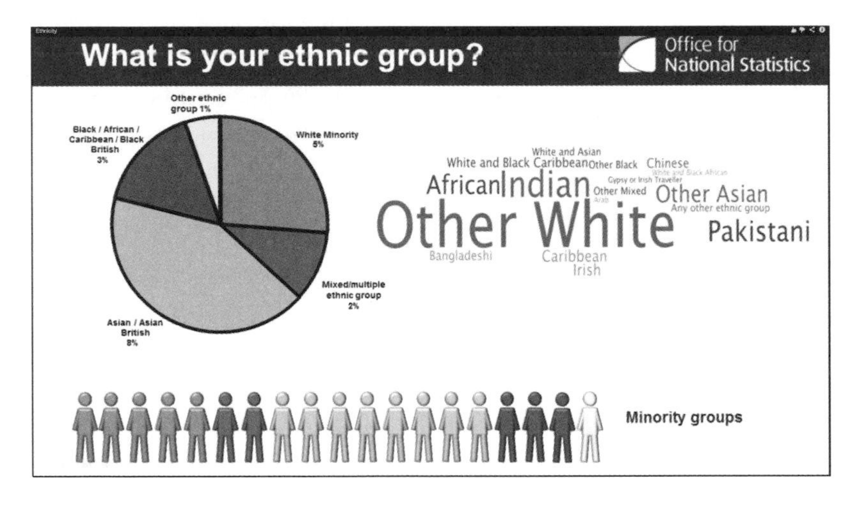

Figure 8.2: Composition of minority ethnic groups in England and Wales: 2011 census

(Source: Office for National Statistics, 2012b, with permission)

The background of older people from black and minority ethnic (BME) communities varies, but patterns of migration that occurred following the Second World War have had a significant influence on the ethnic composition of the current groups aged 65 and over. Craig et al. (2012) write that in the 1940s and 50s there were significant shortages of labour required for postwar construction. War refugees from central Europe found jobs in heavy industry, transport and the new National Health Service (NHS), as did workers recruited from British colonies. Despite their contribution to the British economy and their war service, they were not always welcomed. Racism led to the charging of unfair rents, which resulted in crowded groups of migrants living in large houses. Consequently migrants settled in poorer inner-city areas and so communities grew.

Drawing on census information from 1951 and 1961, Craig et al. (2012) highlight the growth of people from the Indian subcontinent (e.g. India and Pakistan), the Caribbean Islands (e.g. Jamaica), the Far East (e.g. modern-day Malaysia, Indonesia, Myanmar) and West Africa. In 1951 these peoples accounted for 74,500 of the UK population, rising to 336,600 in 1961. As most migrants were of working age, those who settled will be BME elders today. Settled minorities now live in all local authority areas, although the census reveals that the greatest diversity is to be found in large cities. These communities are a mixture of older established groups and newer migrants, including those from forced exits from former colonies such as Uganda in the 1980s. Many have had children and grandchildren born in the UK.

Culture, religion and spiritual beliefs are associated with ethnicity and are factors that impact on perceptions of illness and disability. It is important therefore that nurses understand the changing profile of the population as we are expected *to practise in a caring and sensitive manner that avoids assumptions, supports social inclusion ... and acknowledges diversity* (Nursing and Midwifery Council, 2010). Older people are the largest group of health service users. Care must be tailored to reflect the changing population profile so as to acknowledge and respect differing beliefs and values in the way care is planned and delivered; for example, using a language and manner that allow elders from any ethnic group to make informed choices.

Data concerning the age profile of different ethnic groups are not yet available from the 2011 census. However an experimental data set collected in 2007 by the ONS and reported by Rogers (2010) confirms that the proportion of people from BME communities in the older age groups as a percentage of the population is increasing (Table 8.1).

	Age (years)					
Ethnic group	**65–69**	**70–74**	**75–79**	**80–84**	**85–89**	**Over 90**
White British	2,156.0	1,901.2	1,622.7	1,216.5	748.2	369.9
White minority	101.3	86.9	68.3	51.7	25.2	10.1
Mixed/multiple ethnic group	7.9	6.2	4.5	2.9	1.5	0.7
Asian/Asian British	66.1	52.0	31.3	14.5	7.0	2.5
Black/African/ African Caribbean/ black British	38.5	32.1	19.7	9.6	3.8	1.2
Other	12.1	8.4	5.0	2.5	1.1	0.5

Table 8.1: Older population of England and Wales 2007, by age and ethnic groupings (in thousands)

(Source: data from the Office for National Statistics. Full data set available at: **https://docs.google.com/spreadsheet/ccc?key=0AonYZs4MzlZbdGthMG52UDlxRzYwMzI4aFBuUnFhSUE#gid=0**)

Understanding the terminology

The term ethnicity is often used interchangeably with words such as culture, nationality, religion and race. However meanings differ so some clarification is required.

Activity 8.1 *Reflection*

Take a piece of paper and jot down your response to the question 'who am I?' Try to make a list of ten words.

An outline answer is provided at the end of the chapter.

Our identity can refer to the way we are each unique as well as ways in which we share aspects with others. We frequently draw upon family, nationality and lifestyle to form the mix that helps us to *know who 'we' and 'others' are* (Canton et al., 2008, p. 48). Age and ethnicity and/or culture are defining features of identity for most people. However, concepts such as 'old age' are social constructions, the meaning of which vary over time and between societies. For example, marriage at the age of puberty was acceptable in earlier times in the UK but is now illegal, yet is currently practised in some other countries (Plan UK, 2013). Perceptions of 'marriageable age' are shaped by social, economic and cultural factors prevalent within a particular society at a particular time.

Old age

Similarly, 'old age', 'ethnicity', 'culture', 'race' and 'nationality' are social constructs. Their meaning is learned through the process of primary and secondary socialisation. People learn ways of being and appropriate ways to act in social situations from those involved in their early upbringing (Ritzer, 2007). This is then reinforced by other powerful influences such as education, religion and the media. This process becomes in effect the lens through which we view the world, so much so that it can be difficult to accept that there are different views about the same things held by people socialised in a different society. For example, in most South Asian languages there is no word for dementia. Consequently people from these communities may perceive the signs and symptoms of dementia as just part of 'old age' and therefore not seek help or support until the symptoms become advanced. This leads to lower levels of awareness of dementia in South Asian populations in the UK, and poorer uptake of support and treatment (Moriarty et al., 2011).

Activity 8.2 *Reflection*

Think about 'growing old'. What words would you use to describe the stage in life known as old age?

An outline answer is provided at the end of the chapter.

According to Achenbaum (2005, p. 21), different societies attribute divergent meanings to older age. Our view of ageing often arises from political, social, economic, cultural and demographic factors that reflect a particular society, in a particular place, at a particular time. For example, Chinese and other Asian cultures traditionally confer great respect on older adults as sources of wisdom and knowledge, although this has declined with modernisation and urbanisation as multigenerational households have become less common. In many Western societies a biomedical perspective on ageing dominates: old age is seen as one of loss – loss of faculties, health, social value and social networks.

Case study

Jenny is 75 and was married for 42 years. She was born in Scotland, and moved to South Africa when her husband left the army after the Second World War. Jenny has five children, three of whom are married and have children of their own. Her two daughters moved back to the UK ten years ago and Jenny moved to live nearby in the same town when she was widowed, just over six years ago. Jenny lives alone in a small ground-floor flat leased from a charity for ex-military service personnel and their dependants. She collects two of her grandchildren from school during the school term and cares for them until her daughters (both now divorced) collect them after work. She is the secretary of the local Caledonian Society and arranges social events and fundraising activities. She has diabetes and fell recently, sustaining a venous leg ulcer. She attends the GP surgery to have this dressed using compression bandages once a week.

Jenny views herself as a healthy, active and 'useful' mother and grandmother who also happens to have diabetes. When she visits the practice nurse to have her weekly leg ulcer dressing, she is likely to see this as a temporary situation that she wants to get over quickly and get back to 'normal'. She might feel that her 'age is catching up with her' and therefore the incident might shake her self-confidence. As a practice nurse you will wish to provide nursing care related to the ulcer but equally offer health promotion advice around the avoidance of falls and skin integrity and risk associated with diabetes. Jenny's age will be a factor in your assessment and planned interventions but evidence from the client rather than personal assumptions about older age should be used as your guide for care.

Culture

Culture, ethnicity and 'race' are often used to mean the same thing, although there are significant differences. We are all members of the human race; we all belong to a culture or cultures; we all ascribe ourselves an ethnic origin. The concept of culture is intertwined with ideas about ethnicity and race. Fenton (1999) views culture as a symbolic concept that embodies values, lifestyles, manners, customs, food and dress and is connected with the construction of group boundaries. The danger is that culture can be perceived as simply a (fixed) list of attributes that apply to everybody identified as belonging to a particular culture. Even more problematic is the tendency to attribute behaviours and attitudes to all people from a specific culture on the basis of their perceived group membership. It is all too easy to label people in this way. For example, I am Scottish; on this basis you might think I have red hair, pale skin and blue eyes. You might also believe the jokes and think because I am Scottish, I am mean. Of course this is stereotypical and ridiculous. However Jewish people were 'constructed' by the Nazi party to 'look like rats' and to be inherently enemies of the state, also stereotypical and ridiculous, but a view that led to horrific consequences. Fenton (1999) argues that the association of a culture with a people is a construction and is linked to feelings of nationalism. Indeed, 'culture' tends to be used in everyday language, e.g. Arab culture, Chinese culture, to mean foreign or different, a term used about 'others' to show how 'they' deviate from 'our' cultural norms; this sense of difference sometimes engenders feelings of intolerance.

Ethnicity

Ethnicity is self-assigned. It concerns actual or perceived common ancestry, language and regional or national origin (Fenton, 1999). Ethnic groupings are not fixed, although they are often perceived as if they are, because the word is linked with the notion of racial groupings (see below). Ethnicity is a social construct and so perceptions of ethnic groups are created by society. Linked to this is the concept of essentialism, which is the belief that social differences are determined by biology. This view maintains that ethnicity affects, for example, the character of the person and so a fixed set of characteristics is attributed to a specific ethnic group. This attitude might lead to beliefs such as all Arab women are submissive or all Jewish patients have low pain thresholds. Nurses who hold essentialist views of ethnic groups will tend to make assumptions about individuals based on their perceived group membership. This is not patient-centred and could lead to inappropriate care.

Although people can be grouped by ethnicity (or by gender or class, for that matter), this group affiliation does not define them. So if you meet a new patient and your ethnicity is Asian, for example, you might perceive first that the patient is black, but this is just one aspect of the patient's identity alongside that she is a woman, a mother, a judge, has diabetes and so on. In other words her 'blackness' does not define her.

Ethnicity is only one dimension of social relationships and interacts with others such as gender or age group. However, because ethnicity tends to be judged by others through visual cues like skin colour and facial features, this aspect can have dominance over other facets of identity when meeting new people.

One final issue here is the assumed relationship between religion and ethnicity. The major religions of the world cross many nation states and many ethnic groups; for example a person can be a Muslim who is white British, black or Asian. Equally, 25 per cent of the UK population has no religious belief (ONS, 2013). It is an essentialist perspective to link a particular religion or no religion to a particular ethnic group.

Scenario

Imagine the situation of Abeer, who is 21 years old and was born in Leicester. Abeer has pale skin and blue eyes. She converted to Islam three years ago and wears a jilbab (long outer garment) and hijab (headscarf). Her family rejected her when she converted and decided to marry a British man of Pakistani origin. She worked as a healthcare assistant until she had her first child.

Activity 8.3 *Communication*

What issues might Abeer face when accessing healthcare for her child?

An outline answer is provided at the end of the chapter.

'Race' and racism

The concept of 'race' is based on now discredited scientific theories that humankind could be divided into types based upon differing physical features (Miles and Brown, 2003). 'Race' based on biological difference has no substance in biology, as there are very few genetic differences between so-called racial groups: the degree of variation within racially defined groups is more than the variation between them (Barry and Yuill, 2008).

However, whilst 'race' does not exist, racism does. The historical understanding of race remains a powerful aspect of 'common-sense thinking' and is viewed by some as not only 'true' but 'natural'. Racism embodies the attitude that one race (group perceived as different based on appearance or place of origin) is superior or inferior to another. Therefore racism persists as an influential structural feature of society. Racism is at play when prejudices are used to explain differences; social meanings are attributed to these differences and this leads to exclusionary practices. For example, if the majority of the population assume that Asian people will 'look after their own' in older age (Age Concern, 2010), this may lead to exclusionary practices: people from Asian communities may not be offered postdischarge support following a hospital stay.

Whilst racism is illegal (Equality Act: Home Office, 2010) and discrimination on the grounds of ethnicity/'race' is not tolerated according to the nurses' code of conduct (Nursing and Midwifery Council, 2008b), none the less racism has been evident in the NHS, nursing and nurse education (NSCSHA, 2003; Scammell and Olumide, 2012). Racism is a facet of UK society and as nurses are part of this society, it explains why some may unwittingly practise at times in an exclusionary manner.

Ethnicity, older age and health inequalities

> *How well and how long one lives is powerfully shaped by one's place in the hierarchies around occupation, education, and income.*
> (Graham, 2000, p. 3)

In keeping with similar initiatives across the world, the Equality Act came into force in the UK in 2010. The aim is to provide a single legal framework to tackle disadvantage and discrimination against people on grounds of their membership of certain groups within society; for example, those based on age, ethnicity or religion. According to Scott and Marshall (2009), *Equality exists if everyone has the same or near similar chances to achieve their ends or goals. It is a measure of how fair or equal conditions are at the 'starting gate'.*

Case study

William was born into a family living in the UK in poor housing and as a result suffered chronic respiratory disease and associated illness throughout his first five years. He subsequently performed less well than average at school, due to poor health, and gained low-paid employment. When he reached retirement age he lived only on the state pension. William's life expectancy is likely to be lower than the average.

The notion of 'starting gate' is significant in William's life: we can see that from birth, life chances can be compromised. Scott and Marshall (2009) state that *inequality exists when there are unequal rewards or opportunities for different individuals within a group or groups within a society.* If William had been born into a wealthier family (with greater rewards) they would have been likely to have better housing and the opportunity to pay for additional healthcare (greater opportunities), which might have affected his education and employment chances and ultimately his personal wealth, health and well-being. There is a clear link between poverty and increased experience of ill health (Marmot, 2010). The study of health inequalities involves making comparisons between social groupings such as older age or ethnicity and measures of health outcome, that is to say, the incidence of morbidity (disease) and mortality in different social groups. Health inequality is said to exist when one grouping shows a greater incidence of illness or lowered life expectancy than the average incidence in the total population. Clearly the incidence of morbidity and mortality increases as we age; however if life expectancy is lower and the incidence of mental illness, for example, is higher in certain ethnic groups, this would indicate a health inequality.

Health inequalities and ethnicity

Statistically certain health outcomes have been found to be poorer in specific ethnic groups.

Activity 8.4 — *Critical thinking*

Read the following research summaries of evidence of health inequalities linked to ethnicity compiled for the UK Parliament. Focusing on cardiovascular disease (CVD) or cancer or mental health, suggest some possible explanations for these health inequalities. In writing your notes look at the issues from a holistic perspective.

An outline answer is provided at the end of the chapter.

Research summary

Cardiovascular disease

Men born in South Asia are 50 per cent more likely to have a heart attack or angina than men in the general population. Bangladeshis have the highest rates, followed by Pakistanis, then Indians and other South Asians. By contrast, men born in the Caribbean are 50 per cent more likely to die of stroke than the general population, but they have much lower mortality to coronary heart disease. Classical risk factors like smoking, blood pressure, obesity and cholesterol fail to account for all these ethnic variations, and there is debate about how much they can be explained by socioeconomic factors. Many researchers think that there are biological differences between ethnic groups, and a lot of research has been carried out on the potential mechanisms.

Cancer

Overall, cancer rates tend to be lower in BME groups. For lung cancer, mortality rates are lower in people from South Asia, the Caribbean and Africa, which relates to lower levels of smoking. The highest mortality is found in people from Ireland and Scotland. Mortality from breast cancer is lower for migrant women than for women born in England and Wales. Researchers think this reflects the fact that it takes time to acquire the detrimental lifestyle and other risk factors associated with living in this country.

Mental health

Ethnic differences in mental health are controversial. Most of the data are based on treatment rates, which show that BME people are much more likely to receive a diagnosis of mental illness than the white British. Studies show up to seven times higher rates of new diagnosis of psychosis among black Caribbean people than among the white British. However, surveys on the prevalence of mental illness in the community show smaller ethnic differences. There is evidence of ethnic differences in risk factors that operate before a patient comes into contact with the health services, such as discrimination, social exclusion and urban living. There is also evidence of differences in treatment. For example, black Caribbean and African people are more likely to enter psychiatric care through the criminal justice system than through contact with the health services. Some researchers suggest that psychiatrists diagnose potential symptoms of mental illness differently depending on the ethnicity of the patient.

(Source: Parliamentary Office for Science and Technology (2007) *Postnote: Ethnicity and health*. Available at: **http://www.parliament.uk/documents/post/postpn276.pdf**)

Explanations of variance in health outcome between ethnic groups are complex. For example, there are clear differences in the incidence of CVD (British Heart Foundation, 2010) and cancer rates (National Cancer Intelligence Network and Cancer Research UK, 2009) across ethnic groups. The causative factors are not yet fully understood. In both cases there are a number of non-modifiable factors such as family history and ethnicity. For example, people of white ethnicity have lighter skin tones, increasing their susceptibility to skin cancer. South Asians have low high-density lipoprotein and elevated triglycerides, both of which are linked to the formation of vascular plaques found in CVD. In the latter case, there are also a number of modifiable factors:

- smoking;
- high blood cholesterol;
- high blood pressure;
- uncontrolled diabetes;
- physical inactivity;
- obesity or overweight;
- uncontrolled stress or anger;
- diet high in saturated fat and cholesterol;
- drinking too much alcohol.

These lifestyle factors also go some way to explaining inequalities, particularly when they are related to cultural patterns of living. For example, diets associated with the South Asian community tend to have high levels of salt, ghee and other cooking fats.

Social norms in these communities might also account for the other factors but this does not explain why access to health services is lower in some BME groups. Ahmad and Bradby (2008) argue that marginalisation and racism can impair health-seeking behaviours.

The explanations for mental health inequalities across ethnic groups are even less uncertain but there is no doubt that some groups, notably black Caribbean and black African, are overrepresented in psychiatric hospitals, especially men. This has led to the NHS being described as institutionally racist (NSCSHA, 2003). Indeed, some evidence suggests that marginalised groups such as people from BME communities, lesbian, gay and bisexual and transgender people, Gypsies and Travellers and asylum seekers are perhaps more likely than other groups to face hostility and misunderstanding. As a consequence they are more likely to experience poor mental health.

Mental health problems affect all age groups but dementia is most associated with older age. Psychosocial and spiritual factors appear to impact on the inequalities apparent in accessing specialist services for people with dementia from some BME communities. Moriarty et al. (2011), in a review of the limited research in this area, found lower levels of awareness about dementia as well as a significant stigma about the condition within BME communities. Consequently carers of BME people with dementia may feel reluctant to ask for help.

The government is committed to reducing health inequalities by ensuring that whatever their economic or ethnic background, patients receive the highest possible quality of care (Department of Health, 2008). One way to address this is to review service provision because fair and equal access to services is a right of every NHS patient, regardless of their ethnic origin or where they live in the UK. Sometimes this means providing additional or different kinds of services, for example professional interpreters and patient advocates, to make sure all sectors of society are able to benefit from the NHS.

Becoming aware of our own prejudices

It is perhaps part of the human condition that we look at the world from our own perspective. It is natural to feel more comfortable with people who are 'like us' because we think we understand them better. However it is important that we maintain an open mind about other cultures because nurses provide a universal service to all people. Part of developing an open mind is to become aware of our prejudices and to spot any ethnocentric attitudes. Ethnocentrism is the tendency to evaluate or judge other cultures by the standards of our own, on the premise that our own culture is superior to others (Ritzer, 2007). Ethnocentrism is probably a feature of all cultures and can lead to a biased understanding of others. It may permeate and be reinforced in social institutions such as the family and media and as such is difficult to perceive, particularly if you are a member of a dominant cultural group.

Scenario

Imagine you have a clinical placement in a care home. You have been working with Sue, who is a healthcare assistant. You notice she is rather 'off' with a couple from a South Asian background who came to visit their elderly mother that evening. At your meal break, she mentions that she would never 'put her mother into a home'. Referring to the South Asian couple, she says that they 'should know better and be looking after their mum themselves'. Whilst the same attitude could be applied to all relatives, Sue seems to have different expectations of people from South Asian backgrounds.

As we all have a culture and an ethnic group, we all could experience racism. Equally we are all capable of knowingly or unwittingly engaging in racist behaviour. The most likely manifestation of this is in making assumptions about others, either that they share the same perspective as you or that simply because they seem to belong to an identifiable ethnic group, they will behave according to what you know about that group. Recent research with nurses (Scammell and Olumide, 2012) concerning internationally recruited nurse mentors revealed that essentialist constructions of different cultures were used to explain and justify differences and often to portray these as inferior. For example, referring to a nurse from Ghana, a student stated, 'you can't expect them to be as well trained as they don't have the same standards in their country'. Overt racism was rare but small acts that undermined those perceived as different were frequent. These included arranging off-duty so as not to work with internationally recruited nurse mentors and condoning patient preferences for nurses without foreign accents. This study is an example of the effects of ethnocentrism and, although small, is illustrative of what can happen if nurses make ethnocentric assumptions about the nature of older age.

Perceptions of ageing across cultures

In Activity 8.2 you were asked to note down some words that describe old age. Keep this alongside as you read on. Wray (2003) found in a literature review of the experiences of older women across ethnic and cultural groups that the focus was placed upon the problems associated with growing old. Furthermore, whilst concepts such as quality of life and successful ageing were often used, these appeared to be culturally defined from the perspective of the researchers and as such overwhelmingly reflected the assumptions that underpin Western medicine. Healthy ageing, for example, was linked to autonomy, independence and perceptions about dis/empowerment; it was assumed that all older women would value these attributes in older age.

Wray (2003) then conducted a qualitative study involving South Asian, African-Caribbean, British-Irish and Dominican older women from Christian, Sikh and Muslim backgrounds, focused on their perceptions of later life. All shared the view that good health was central to quality of life in older age. Rather than focusing on deficiencies in older age, the women concentrated on what they could do and adapted accordingly. Some women had experienced racism, particularly in their youth, and this they argued made them strong and able to cope with life's struggles. Some relied on the physical and psychological support of their cultural group and maintained their sense of control through this lifestyle choice rather than viewing this as dependence. Respect from others also provided a sense of well-being, as did the adoption of new roles in the care of grandchildren and the social interactions related to religious beliefs and practices.

Differences and similarities: four perspectives

A central message of this chapter is that nurses need to understand cultural differences but the study by Wray (2003) teaches us to avoid assumptions in our interactions with those we perceive to be different. Each older person is an expert on themselves and you should tap into this to provide culturally appropriate care.

Activity 8.5 — *Critical thinking*

When caring for older people, nurses who were brought up outside the UK will have certain perceptions about care for older people. Four brief narratives from students from abroad but studying nursing in the UK are provided in the case studies below. As you read them, identify the issues they highlight about care for older people in their home country. Illustrate this in the form of a mind map.

An outline answer is provided at the end of the chapter.

Case studies

Ida from Cameroon

In my country, deaths from HIV/AIDS are high, leaving many grandparents to bring up their grandchildren. This can be hard but they feel they are doing something useful as they get older. It is expected that children and grandchildren look after their grandparents but young people are moving to the cities to find work, leaving many older people on their own with little money because not many get pensions. People use herbal remedies a lot. Religion is very important. Older people prefer to go to Christian missionary hospitals because they feel they are cared for with compassion and according to their beliefs.

Jitka from the Czech Republic

Older people are treated with great respect; younger people give them their seat on the bus and we always address them formally. Older people are seen as wise and should be listened to. To be touched by a stranger is not acceptable except when this is necessary for hospital care. There is little state-funded care and the hospitals for the old are feared because people go there to die. So people try to stay at home and pay for nurses but cost is a big worry as many younger family members choose to work abroad and aren't around to care for them.

Pooja from Nepal

We are expected to care for older family members and, if we live abroad, to send money home. Communities are close and so if an older person does not have children, other family members will care for them or even neighbours. Elders are highly respected and are always addressed by their family name, like Grandmother, and even if they are not your family, as Aunt or whatever. A stranger using their first name would cause great offence. Older people like their family to be involved with care and to have people they know around them. Religion is important and people use spiritual healers when doctors can't help them.

Irina from Romania

Unless they are rich, older people in my country go into hospital as a last resort as the care is not compassionate. The wards are crowded and people feel unsafe and lonely. Families try to care for them if they can as older people often provide child care so that the younger adults can work. But dementia is becoming a big problem because it gets to the point where it is unsafe for someone with dementia to care for young children. So they have to go into hospital because they can't help at home and their children have to work to care for their own children.

The ideas described in the case studies may influence expectations of older people and their families about care in the UK. However, looking at these accounts, regardless of an individual's place of origin, similar concepts seem to underpin opinions about good care in later life. Do not assume you know what the concept of respect means to an individual, for example, as shown in language or manner used to address someone.

A number of guides exist to help nurses understand different religious and cultural beliefs (Help the Aged/RCN, 2008). These are useful resources but it is difficult to know about every cultural group in depth. Empathetic communication skills will enable nurses to make the initial connection; in the example of what to call someone, the most respectful solution is simply to ask. 'Hello, I am a nurse and my name is Jude. Would you like me to call you Mrs Satish?' If we base care around fundamental values about what it means to be human we will meet the needs of all patients, including those who are ethnically or culturally different from ourselves.

Responding to cultural diversity in the healthcare context: the humanising values framework

> *Act as if what you do makes a difference. It does.*
> (William James, philosopher)

Nurses aim to promote health and well-being, minimise distress and suffering, enable people to manage disease or disability and, when death is likely, to maintain well-being until the end of life. But a number of recent reports have highlighted poor healthcare. The Report of the Mid Staffordshire NHS Foundation Trust Public Inquiry (Francis, 2013) described significant shortcomings. The care of older people attracted considerable criticism as numerous examples were cited where basic human needs were not met. Likewise, the serious case review into care of clients with learning disabilities at the Winterbourne View Hospital (Flynn, 2012a) shockingly demonstrated the impact of a culture where staff were permitted to treat a group of people as 'objects', denying their humanity.

Some older people with physical or mental health problems or those with learning difficulties may feel vulnerable. This is worse where the person also has differences in communication or lifestyle, such as some people from BME communities. Nursing education based on a humanising values framework has at its centre a genuine and empathetic relationship with service users and carers (Scammell et al., 2012). Whilst excellent knowledge and technical competence are essential to professional care giving, addressing the human dimensions of care is also crucially important. The humanising values framework (Galvin and Todres, 2012) can be used to guide our nursing care to focus on what is important to us as human beings; it helps you value and respond to the experience of the service user as a first priority. Within this framework, the ethnicity of the client and associated values and belief systems are viewed as important aspects of identity that will influence an individual's experience of health, illness and care.

Galvin and Todres (2012) argue that explicitly focusing on the experience or 'lifeworld' of service users and carers makes care authentic. By holding at the centre of our work the things that 'make us feel human' rather than concentrating on the medical diagnosis or 'routine' care, nurses can practise humanly sensitive care. Understanding the potentially humanising and dehumanising elements (Table 8.2) in caring systems and interactions enables us to care for everyone more effectively, including people of a different ethnicity to ourselves.

Forms of humanisation	Forms of dehumanisation
Insiderness	Objectification
Agency	Passivity
Uniqueness	Homogenisation
Togetherness	Isolation
Sense making	Loss of meaning
Personal journey	Loss of personal journey
Sense of place	Dislocation
Embodiment	Reductionist body

Table 8.2: Dimensions of the humanising values framework

(Source: adapted from Galvin and Todres, 2012)

Application to practice

The principles that underpin excellent nursing care apply regardless of your ethnicity or your patient's. However we tend to view the world from our own perspective. A nurse who uses the humanising values framework tries to imagine what it is like for the person experiencing a condition or care, that is, from the patient's perspective.

Scenario

On the medical ward is an 80-year-old woman named Rabeea Malik. Mrs Malik is Muslim, born in Pakistan and she moved to the UK over 40 years ago. She was admitted in the night following a fall at home. She was diagnosed with a chest infection; she is also dehydrated and confused. She has two adult children and three grandchildren. Her husband died 18 months ago. Mrs Malik lives with her eldest son who works night shifts as a bus driver. After her fall, she pressed her personal alarm and this alerted her younger son (who lives 30 minutes away with his wife, mother-in law and adult children) to come to the house, from where he called an ambulance. Mrs Malik is scheduled to go to radiology for a chest X-ray shortly.

Activity 8.6 — *Decision making*

You arrive for duty in a medical ward and have been allocated to care for Mrs Malik. Make a brief list of care priorities and anticipated nursing actions for the next few hours.

An outline answer is provided at the end of the chapter.

When asked to care for a patient of whatever ethnicity, certain priorities will be identical. You will need to familiarise yourself with the patient documentation. On first meeting Mrs Malik, you will use your knowledge of the signs, symptoms and management of chest infections in older people to make a holistic appraisal of the person in front of you. Apart from observations using all your senses, your main tool will be communication. You will need to introduce yourself and ask what name the patient would like you to use to address her. You will explain the need for assessment. Whilst talking you will need to assess understanding. Do not make assumptions. Given the history of confusion, understanding might be compromised by delirium associated with the infection and/or limited understanding of English. As when meeting all patients for the first time, your role is to make a genuine connection through a caring and compassionate approach in order to allay anxieties and fears. All your care should involve the patient in whatever way possible as well as the family when appropriate and with the patient's consent.

You will have identified a number of nursing actions to take in Activity 8.6. Cultural beliefs are most likely to influence how you might put these plans into action rather than change significantly the fundamentals of care offered to any clients with similar medical needs. The humanising values framework is useful to consider not so much what you do as a nurse when working with culturally diverse clients, but how you do it. We now go on to consider all eight dimensions of the humanising values framework with practical examples of how this affects your nursing practice.

Dimension 1: Insiderness/objectification

This dimension highlights the need to think about care from the perspective of the person experiencing it rather than treating the person like an object or set of tasks linked with a diagnosis. Many people of Muslim faith prefer to be washed by someone of the same gender or in this case a close female relative. This task may need to be delayed until appropriate staff or family members are available. Such a delay would prevent objectification, where completing a task took precedence over the patient's preferences.

See the further reading and useful websites at the end of the chapter for resources which will help.

Dimension 2: Agency/passivity

Agency reflects an NHS priority to make patients agents in their care; that is, to promote genuine choice for patients both in terms of accessing care and having a say in decisions about care; passivity is about feeling like care is 'done to you'. However genuine, choice can only be made by individuals who are informed and understand what this means and their rights in the process. It is important to remember that a good understanding of everyday English (as a second language) will not necessarily mean a good understanding of medical English. And of course all patients, worried about their illness and probably disoriented, will have difficulty understanding all you say. Do not assume everyone can read and write English or any other language (Age Concern, 2010). Advocacy is a major way to facilitate agency where understanding is impaired for whatever reason and helps prevent unintended discrimination.

Dimension 3: Uniqueness/homogenisation

Older people are not a homogeneous group and neither are all people of South Asian ethnicity. Whilst Mrs Malik and her immediate family may live according to the typical life ways associated with people of the Muslim faith, this cannot be assumed. For example, men are perceived as protectors of women and as such to be consulted in major decisions over health matters. However, changing family structures and exposure to other cultural values in generations born in the UK mean this cannot be assumed. It is important therefore to ensure interpretation services are used when required rather than to rely on family members for this so that the patient can make an informed choice, even if that choice is to defer to her son.

Dimension 4: Togetherness/isolation

We found in Activity 8.5 that companionship, feeling in control and being valued were important facets of care for older people. The basis of the togetherness/isolation dimension recognises the importance of feeling in contact with people who understand your ways of being. Feeling unwell and in hospital makes people feel isolated, without control over decisions about the smallest of things, as well as purposeless. When facing problems with health and well-being, most of us value the support of others. Encourage participation in care (if desired by the patient) from family members and visits from people from worship communities or community groups; this can help people to retain a sense of who they are whilst dealing with the demands of their illness.

Dimension 5: Sense making/loss of meaning

Many of us take our health for granted and when we become ill it can be difficult to make sense of what is happening. You may assume nurses know what is best for the patient based on their expertise but try to understand the situation from the patient's perspective. In long-term life-limiting conditions, ask patients what is the most important thing for them to feel better at a particular time; this can be both empowering and empathetic. Facilitating someone to practise his or her faith may provide much comfort. For example, Muslims and Christians, among others, seek God's help to overcome illness through prayer; to facilitate ritual washing and appropriate positioning for Muslims would reflect compassionate care.

Dimension 6: Personal journey/loss of personal journey

Facing illness and perhaps coming into the care of health professionals is one small part of the person's total life journey. This journey has shaped who the individual is now and helps the person to deal with new challenges. Acknowledging and working with personal history, particularly in situations of cognitive impairment, helps people to retain their sense of identity. Mrs Malik (in the case study) appears to have delirium but taking note of significant names and places and perhaps previous work or place of residence would be helpful links with her personal journey for staff to use when family or community members were not present. Life-story books are an extension of this; according to Moriarty et al. (2011), these are a powerful tool in preserving identity and communication with people with dementia in general, but especially with people from BME communities.

Dimension 7: Sense of place/dislocation

Home for most of us is where we feel comfortable and is heavily influenced by cultural patterns. Food has an important place in our sense of home – what we eat, when we eat and how we eat as well as food associated with celebratory events. Hospital admission is a dislocation but a sense of place like home and the comfort this engenders can be created to some extent through the provision of culturally acceptable dietary choices. This is a vital part of nursing care, as Mrs Malik will require a nutritious diet to fight infection. Muslims consider the left hand to be unclean and so the right hand should be used for feeding and administering medication.

Dimension 8: Embodiment/reductionism

Whilst knowing nothing about cultures that are different from one's own is unacceptable, so also is making assumptions about 'other' cultures based on stereotypical descriptions of what 'they' do. This would be an example of reductionism, when the complexity of people from one ethnic group, for example, is reduced to a 'recipe book' of practices applied to all people of that group. Embodiment is about trying to understand and acknowledge the central essence of the person. This is fundamental to person-centred care. You may find it difficult to connect with some people; through sensitive communication and perhaps intuition you might hit on something that really matters to the person and that becomes the key to your relationship.

Summary points to guide practice

The humanising values framework highlights ways to think about care from the perspective of the person experiencing it. All of us would want compassionate, respectful and dignified care, regardless of our age or ethnicity, but also care that acknowledges differences inherent with our age and ethnicity. Needs are universal but the solutions to address them may be somewhat different.

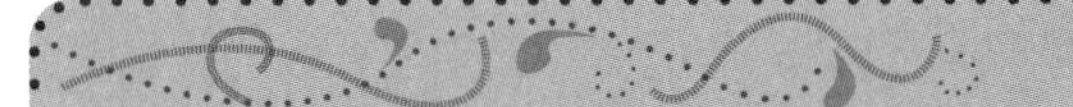

Chapter summary

This chapter has considered the growth in cultural diversity of the UK older population and the implications for care. Terminology used when considering cultural diversity were explained and related to attitudes towards people who are perceived as different. The nature of health inequalities in relation to ethnicity was explored, including the link to poorer physical and mental health outcome. Different perceptions of ageing across ethnic groups were considered and, whilst differences were apparent, so were many similarities. It was suggested that providing culturally appropriate care required an approach that valued the humanity of people. This humanising values framework encourages the nurse to consider client need from the perspective of the person requiring care and to use this insight alongside professional knowledge and skills to provide care that is both compassionate and culturally sensitive.

Activities: brief outline answers

Activity 8.1

Typically we draw upon social institutions and groupings to describe ourselves. The answer to: 'who am I' might include:

- your place within a family structure or your employment status;
- your nationality or culture or religion or favourite leisure pursuit;
- your age, gender, class, ethnicity or religion.

Activity 8.2

advancing years, autumn of life, debility, declining years, decrepitude, dotage, elderliness, evening of life, feebleness, geriatrics, golden years, infirmity, longevity, oldness, retirement age, second childhood, senescence, senility, seniority

(Source: **http://thesaurus.com/browse/old+age**)

Do you think that this social construction of older age seems to reflect a perspective of older age as a period of decline?

Activity 8.3

Healthcare professionals may make assumptions about Abeer and her child based on her ethnicity or based on her apparent religious affiliation. The key to effective care when people are able to communicate for themselves is not to make any assumptions but to ask and seek clarification before doing what you think the person wants.

Activity 8.4

Explanations of health inequalities are multifactorial and therefore complex. Depending on which area you selected, you may have highlighted the following issues:

- physical: biological and genetic factors; effects of environmental pollution; lack of exercise;
- psychological: lifestyle stress, fear of and actual racism; misinterpretation of behaviour; limited language skills affecting access to and understanding of health advice;
- social: lifestyles where high-fat, high-salt, high-sugar diets are the cultural norm; excessive alcohol consumption; smoking; social isolation; social exclusion;
- spiritual: attributions of meaning of health and illness affecting help-seeking behaviour; reliance on spiritual leaders for health guidance; exclusive use of complementary medicines.

Activity 8.5

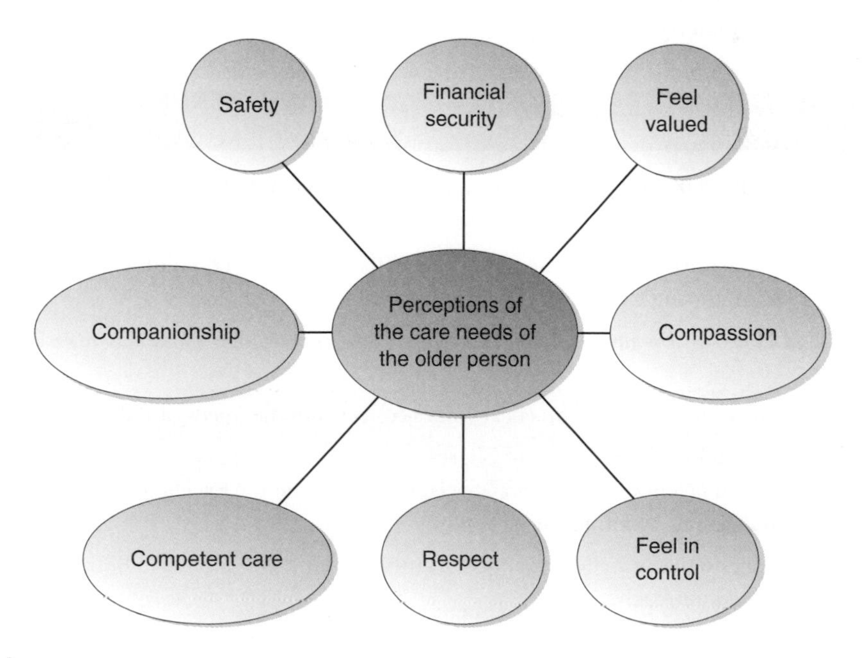

Figure 8.3

Activity 8.6

When asked to care for a patient of whatever ethnicity, certain priorities are identical:

- Physical assessment and interventions: humidified oxygen, availability of suction, collect sputum specimens, encourage expectoration; ensure hydration – care of IV infusion, encourage diet and oral fluids and establish preferences; sit upright, encourage mobility between bed and chair, encourage leg movements in bed; monitor urinary output, collect midstream specimen; take observations – skin condition, temperature, pulse, blood pressure, respirations; administer prescribed medications – IV antibiotics, antipyretics.
- Psychosocial: check for signs of discomfort, anxiety or distress; cognitive assessment, including understanding and language; introduce yourself and ask about the patient's preferred name; state your role and explain what you are doing and why. Keep touch at an instrumental level. Ask how the patient feels and what her biggest difficulty is at present. Ask if she wishes to see a spiritual advisor. Explain forthcoming X-ray.

Useful websites

http://www.ageconcernyorkshireandhumber.org.uk/BME

This website, developed by Age Concern, includes a video about a project for BME elders, aimed at increasing access to health and social care services.

http://www.diversiton.com/downloads/checkUp.pdf

Check Up! A guide to the special healthcare needs of ethnic-religious minority communities is a short guide for nursing.

http://www.nursingtimes.net/nursing-with-dignity-part-8-islam/206284.article

This resource might be useful if you are unfamiliar with life ways associated with people of the Muslim faith.

http://www.ons.gov.uk/ons/rel/census/2011-census/key-statistics-for-local-authorities-in-england-and-wales/video-summary-ethnicity.html

This website is linked to a short video that summarises ethnicity statistics from the 2011 census for England and Wales in an easily understood format.

Further reading

Burnard, P and Gill, P (2009) *Culture, Communication and Nursing: A multicultural guide.* Harlow: Pearson Education.

This is a useful book that focuses on some important differences between cultures and their impact on communication within nursing care.

Help the Aged/RCN (2008) *Dignity on the Ward: Working with older people from ethnic minorities.* London: Help the Aged.

This booklet is one in a series of short, practical guides concerning the needs of BME groups.

Moriarty, J, Sharif, N and Robinson, J (2011) SCIE research briefing 35. *Black and Minority Ethnic People with Dementia and Their Access to Support and Services.* Social Care Institute for Excellence. Available at: **http://www.scie.org.uk/publications/briefings/briefing35**

This briefing paper provides an excellent overview of attitudes towards dementia in BME communities and issues around access and outreach.

Chapter 9
Social isolation and loneliness in later life

Eleanor Jack

NMC Standards for Pre-registration Nursing Education

Domain 1: Professional values

2. All nurses must practise in a holistic, non-judgmental, caring and sensitive manner that avoids assumptions, supports social inclusion; recognises and respects individual choice; and acknowledges diversity. Where necessary, they must challenge inequality, discrimination and exclusion from access to care.
3. All nurses must support and promote the health, wellbeing, rights and dignity of people, groups, communities and populations. These include people whose lives are affected by ill health, disability, ageing, death and dying. Nurses must understand how these activities influence public health.
4. All nurses must work in partnership with service users, carers, families, groups, communities and organisations.

Domain 2: Communication and interpersonal skills

1. All nurses must build partnerships and therapeutic relationships through safe, effective and non-discriminatory communication. They must take account of individual differences, capabilities and needs.

Domain 3: Nursing practice and decision making

3. All nurses must carry out comprehensive, systematic nursing assessments that take account of relevant physical, social, cultural, psychological, spiritual, genetic and environmental factors, in partnership with service users and others through interaction, observation and measurement.
5. All nurses must understand public health principles, priorities and practice in order to recognise and respond to the major causes and social determinants of health, illness and health inequalities.

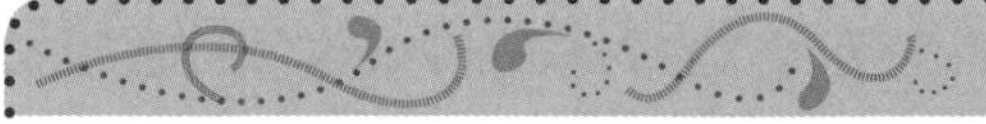

NMC Essential Skills Clusters (ESCs)

This chapter will support the following ESCs:

Cluster: Care, compassion and communication

2. People can trust the newly registered graduate nurse to engage in person centred care empowering people to make choices about how their needs are met when they are unable to meet them themselves.
3. People can trust the newly registered graduate nurse to respect them as individuals and strive to help them preserve their dignity at all times.
5. People can trust the newly registered graduate nurse to engage with them in a warm, sensitive and compassionate way.
6. People can trust the newly registered graduate nurse to engage therapeutically and actively listen to their needs and concerns, responding using skills that are helpful, providing information that is clear, accurate, meaningful and free from jargon.

Chapter aims

After reading this chapter you will be able to:

- describe what is meant by social isolation and loneliness;
- describe the negative impacts on health and well-being that social isolation and loneliness may have on the older person;
- identify person-centred strategies that will enable you to harness older people's ability to establish and maintain meaningful social relationships and friendships;
- recognise the role that the nurse can have as a facilitator and enabler in working with older people.

Introduction

As has been mentioned in earlier chapters, the literature suggests that a good quality of later life is influenced not only by our ability to maintain autonomy and independence (World Health Organization, 2007) but also by our having meaningful social relationships.

Activity 9.1 — *Reflection*

What do you think is meant by 'meaningful' social relationships? Write down what you think this means and then consider whether you have meaningful social relationships in your own life.

As this is a personal reflection, no outline answer is supplied.

Before you begin reading this chapter, it is important to remember that the majority of older people enjoy good mental health and have a strong sense of well-being, as has been articulated in other chapters (Lee, 2006).

There is increasing policy interest nationally, and internationally, seeking to maintain older people's well-being, with a renewed focus on services and practice that support and promote older people's quality of life. Strengthening social networks, supporting social engagement and reducing social isolation and loneliness in particular have been identified as ways of improving older people's quality of life and well-being (Cattan et al., 2003, 2005; Bowling and Gabriel, 2007).

The Social Care Institute for Excellence (2012) states: *As the UK's population rapidly ages, the issue of acute loneliness and social isolation is one of the biggest challenges facing our society.* They go on to highlight that contemporary research suggests that, amongst those aged over 65, between 5 and 16 per cent report feeling lonely and 12 per cent feel isolated. The number of older adults feeling isolated and lonely is expected to increase in the coming years.

As has been suggested in earlier chapters, older people themselves recognise that having good social networks and relationships is important for their mental health (Social Care Institute for Excellence, 2007), as well as keeping engaged in purposeful activity (Reed et al., 2003). This factor is important for you as a nurse to consider within your practice. You will already be familiar with many of the nursing philosophies, theories and models that inform your practice when caring for clients so that their autonomy and independence are maintained as they move towards recovery and well-being, but have you ever considered your role in facilitating the social relationships in their lives and the reason why you should be doing so?

This chapter will describe the commonly used definitions of social isolation and loneliness and explore the experience of social isolation and loneliness from the older person's perspective. The latter is important as research on this subject frequently fails to seek and listen to the voice of the older person (Stanley et al., 2010).

We will look at the negative physical and mental health impacts that experiencing social isolation can have on well-being, as well as considering how society may contribute to social isolation through exclusion by stigmatising and discriminating against older people.

Finally, the chapter will expand on the value that older people place on having friendships, focusing on the positive impacts that they have on their well-being, crucially, in reducing social isolation. This will enable you to recognise and address social isolation with older people by identifying and harnessing their skills, knowledge and experience to manage and develop their own strategies for maintaining well-being, in this case to develop and maintain meaningful social relationships and friendships. This collaborative approach is different from the traditional 'needs/problem-based' approach to care for the older person and it is important to recognise the role that you, as a nurse, can have as a facilitator and enabler in working with older people.

Definitions of social isolation and loneliness

The reflection below will help you to consider possible definitions for social isolation and loneliness.

Activity 9.2 — *Critical thinking*

- If a social worker said to you that a community mental health team client was socially isolated, what do you think the social worker meant by this term?
- If a volunteer at a local community church club for older people mentioned to you that a member seemed lonely, what do think was meant by this term?
- Do you think the terms social isolation and loneliness have the same meaning?
- Do you think social isolation and loneliness mean the same to everyone?

An outline answer is provided at the end of the chapter.

The terms loneliness, social isolation and living alone are used interchangeably within the research literature, although they are three distinct (but linked) concepts. Living alone – living in one-person accommodation without others – is the simplest and most objective term to measure.

Loneliness

Loneliness refers to how individuals feel about their level and quality of social contact and engagement; for example, do they feel they see or have meaningful contact with others enough? De Jong-Gierveld (1987) suggests that loneliness can be described as negatively perceived social isolation. It is perhaps easier defined as *the unpleasant experience that occurs when a person's network of social relationships is deficient in some important way, either quantitatively or qualitatively* (Peplau and Perlman, 1982, p. 31). The authors are suggesting either that a person may feel that he or she does not have enough people in his or her life, or, that there are enough people, but there is a lack of meaningful engagement with them.

Emotional isolation and social isolation can be viewed as two aspects of loneliness in older people. Van-Baarsen et al. (2001) and Vincenzi and Grabosky (1987) define social isolation as a deficiency in social integration, and emotional isolation as a deficiency in intimacy and attachments. Figure 9.1 draws together these concepts.

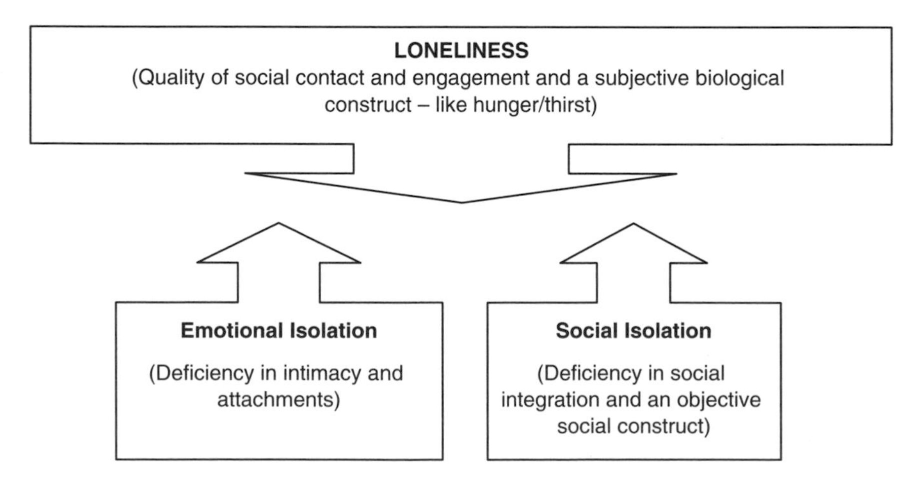

Figure 9.1: Dimensions of loneliness and social isolation

(Source: adapted from the work of van Baarsen et al. (2001) and Vincenzi and Grabosky (1987).)

Social isolation

Any of us may feel lonely and/or isolated at various points in our lives. However, for most of us, these are relatively short-lived feelings which we have (or develop) the external support and internal resilience to cope with. However, for some people, the experience is much more problematic – *difficult life changes or circumstances can bring on a feeling of all-encompassing loneliness/isolation which can become progressively harder to alleviate, leading to feeling stuck in a loop of negative thoughts and behaviours* (Hole, 2011, p. 5).

Although often discussed in the same context as loneliness, social isolation differs in that it concerns an objective description of a situation where there are few recorded or reported actual contacts with other people. That means that it is usually a description of circumstances, such as where an individual has minimal contact with others and/or a generally low level of involvement in community life. Therefore when thinking about social isolation as a concept, we consider that it is usually measured by the number, type and duration of contacts between individuals and the wider social environment, that is, measuring an individual's social network. Other network-related indicators sometimes included are living arrangements (e.g. living alone), availability of a confidant and community involvement (Boldy and Grenade, 2008).

It is important to note that, while a person with a very small number of contacts can be said to be socially isolated, loneliness is not always directly connected to such social isolation. Crucially, socially isolated people may not be lonely and lonely people may not be socially isolated – have you ever felt lonely in a crowd or within a relationship? Conceptualising in this way and from Figure 9.1, it can be seen that loneliness and isolation are not the same, although clearly linked. Therefore, to be successful in tackling loneliness, social isolation also needs to be considered (Age UK, 2010a, p. 3). When you wonder whether an older person feels lonely or not, it is also good to think about improving existing opportunities for social contacts.

It is important to recognise that the literature suggests that older people do not seem to differentiate between social isolation and loneliness according to the definitions; it is their personal experiences rather than the actual definition that matters to them.

Can being alone be healthy?

Critical thinking leads us to consider whether there is another view regarding social isolation and loneliness. Albert Einstein suggested that *I live in that solitude which is painful in youth, but delicious in the years of maturity.*

Activity 9.3 — ***Critical thinking***

What do you think Einstein may have meant by that statement? Do you think there are positive benefits to be had from periods of solitude?

An outline answer is provided at the end of the chapter.

There are benefits to be had from chosen periods of solitude. They offer a chance for reflection on our life, and perhaps reconnecting with what is important for our well-being, e.g. a solitary activity (reading) or following important spiritual pursuits (exercise, meditation, being with animals, linking with nature or religious activities). Importantly, however, it needs to be noted that this solitude is chosen – the individual has a choice. Those who feel lonely or isolated have no choice but to live in solitude. Consider, for a moment, others who also have no choice but to live in solitude, for example, prisoners who are sentenced to solitary confinement as a punishment or for their own safety. There is an abundance of research which confirms the harmful effects of such a sentence (Haney, 2003, p. 130). How often have you heard people saying that they feel *like a prisoner in their own home* as they feel unable to leave? Just like prisoners, they suffer the same harmful experiences.

Griffin (2010) suggests that loneliness is a universal emotion and that it is in actual fact simply *a healthy prompt to look for social contact.* Talking about these feelings helps people feel that they are not alone in their loneliness, or in some way 'abnormal', and that it is in fact a feeling that can be managed and even changed. People who believe in 'putting on a brave face' often find it difficult to admit that they are isolated or lonely as they feel a sense of shame and believe that there is some stigma attached to experiencing loneliness. One in three people would be embarrassed to admit to being lonely (Griffin, 2010).

As a nurse, through your therapeutic relationships with clients, you are in an ideal position not only to assess whether clients are at risk of being socially isolated, but also to establish through talking with them whether or not they feel lonely. In considering the positive dimensions of solitude mentioned above, you can begin what may be a difficult conversation from an empowering positive perspective.

> *Language ... has created the word 'loneliness' to express the pain of being alone. And it has created the word 'solitude' to express the glory of being alone.*
> (Tillich, 2002)

What factors contribute to an older person feeling lonely or isolated?

Before we consider the factors identified in the research literature, do the activity outlined below as this will help you identify for yourself some of the most common factors.

Activity 9.4 — *Reflection*

Make a note of how many people in the last 24 hours you have:

1. spoken with:
   (a) in person;
   (b) on the telephone/cellphone;
   (c) via online webcam/videolink.

(continued)

continued ...

2. written to or received:
   (a) letters;
   (b) texts;
   (c) online e-mail.

3. communicated with via other social media, e.g. Twitter, Facebook.
4. touched/had physical contact with.

As this is based on personal experience, no outline answer is supplied.

This activity will have given you an idea as to how much daily contact you have with others.

Now explore your notes in greater detail by doing the following further reflection.

Activity 9.5 *Reflection*

Having looked at your list, what was the context for all these contacts? For example, was it related to work, society (news or entertainment), planning social/recreational activities, health, chatting with friends, family or partner?

Now consider the following:

- How much technology do you use for communication?
- Is this technology easy or difficult to master?
- Is it expensive to use regularly?
- Do you have to travel to meet up with people?

As this is a reflection, no outline answer is supplied.

Having thought about social contacts, you now may have some understanding as to why an older person can become isolated or feel lonely.

Generally, the universal process of ageing may see a person progressively adapting to his or her changing life and personal circumstances, such as retirement, bereavement or relocation (often into needs-identified accommodation). At the same time, there may be changes in a person's health which require adaptation, e.g. impaired cognition (impacts of dementia/stroke), hearing/sight changes, altered mobility (Hammill, 2009) or incontinence (Nicholson, 2012). It is emerging changes such as these that can lead older people to experience loneliness or social isolation as they may need to modify, or even surrender, lifelong activities that previously ensured meaningful engagement with others.

Other risk factors include a lack of access to private transport, minimal or no contact with friends and family, and living alone as well as low income. Chronic physical or mental health conditions may also contribute to the older person becoming isolated or lonely.

The Cornell Institute for Translational Research on Aging suggests the following factors as contributing to social isolation and loneliness.

- Role loss: The loss of intimate relationships with spouse and friends due to bereavement and the loss of key social roles such as employment or volunteering.
- Living alone: In Western society, both men and women have become less likely to live with relatives other than a partner. This trend has been described as a major demographic shift for the twentieth/twenty-first century.
- Bereavement: Whilst women are more likely to live alone in the later years, partially due to widowhood, they often maintain larger social networks than older men who live alone. It is suggested that men tend to rely primarily on their spouse for social support and, as they age, tend not to rebuild networks after losing their partner.
- Health changes and challenges: Individuals with (perhaps chronic) physical or mental conditions, e.g. heart failure, depression and/or dementia, may not only present issues in themselves but can lower confidence in themselves as individuals and their abilities to get out and mix with others. Discrimination and stigma for these physical or mental health conditions can also affect how the older person integrates with the wider society.
- Poverty: Those older people on a low or restricted income may suffer most from social isolation and loneliness. Having little money can affect the ability to travel and access transport and participate in social activities themselves. The current economic recession has seen the cost of everyday living rise and the closure of many amenities that older people may have been able to access as part of their social life, e.g. post offices, clubs, pubs and libraries, as well as a significant reduction in the availability of public transport.
- Ageing of the Baby Boomers: It is thought that the generation called Baby Boomers (considered as a person who was born during the post-Second World War baby boom between the years 1946 and 1964) will experience social isolation or loneliness given their identified lower rates of marriage, higher levels of divorce and fewer children (Easterlin, 1987; Macunovich, 1995). Female Baby Boomers gave birth to, on average, fewer than two children who survived to age 40 years (Easterlin, 1987; Easterlin et al., 1990). The experienced higher rates of divorce often result in weakened intergenerational bonds, lower contact with children and presumably less emotional support in old age (Uhlenberg and Miner, 1996).

Many of the above factors can be embraced under the umbrella term social exclusion. Social exclusion is defined as *an experience characterised by poverty and the lack of access to social networks, activities and services that results in a poor quality of life* (Bartram, 2005). In the UK, 1.2 million people over 50 are severely excluded, and a woman over the age of 85 is six times more likely to be severely excluded than a woman aged between 65 and 69. One in five people over 80 living alone are severely excluded, and men over 80 living alone are 11 times more likely to be lonely than men over 80 who are living with a partner (Age Concern, 2008). Those aged 50–64 are eight times more likely to be severely socially excluded if they rent their home privately than if they own it or pay a mortgage, with over half of the homes that are privately rented by the over-50s being considered as non-decent (Age Concern, 2008).

The Social Exclusion Unit (Bartram, 2005) highlights that social exclusion can come about due to many circumstances, such as lack of access to leisure, poverty, chronic illness (mental or physical), carer responsibilities, social isolation, fear of crime, age discrimination, lack of appropriate transport, lack of information, services not responsive to needs of users and a lack of accessible information. Those older people from different cultural, religious or ethnic backgrounds (e.g. older gypsies and travellers), as well as those with a learning disability, prisoners, refugees and asylum seekers are already facing existing multiple exclusion factors as they age.

Furthermore, as mentioned earlier, ageism, stigma and discrimination also add to the experience of social exclusion and therefore add to the experience of social isolation and loneliness for the older person, as we have seen in earlier chapters. Indeed, society is predominantly ageist and people are less valued, less visible and more powerless as they get older (see Chapter 6).

The promotion of social inclusion features prominently in current policy across government departments. For example, the Equality Act 2010 came into being as a legal framework to protect the rights of individuals and promote equal opportunity for all. Other relevant policies include *Inclusion Health: Improving primary care for socially excluded people* (Department of Health, 2010a), *Tackling Health Inequalities: 10 years on* (Department of Health, 2009a), *Working Together – UK national action plan on social inclusion 2008–2010* (Department for Work and Pensions, 2008) and *Fair Society, Healthy Lives – The Marmot review* (Department of Health, 2010b). Making Every Adult Matter is a coalition of four national charities which represent over 1,600 front-line organisations formed to influence policy and services for adults facing multiple needs and exclusions, and as an organisation it provides reports to engage with and influence government policy. The Royal College of Nursing website (see useful websites at the end of the chapter) has further information and links on addressing social inclusion for our clients.

The government white paper, *Our Health, Our Care, Our Say* (Department of Health, 2006) acknowledges that social exclusion, isolation and loneliness contribute to the incidence of mental illness, particularly depression.

Given the many variables that may contribute to social exclusion, Bartram (2005) highlights that in addressing social exclusion 'one size' will not fit all, as older people are not (as has been mentioned often in this book already) a homogeneous group. Each older person is an individual with a wealth of experiences and a different life narrative to share and therefore will require the sensitive input of you as a nurse, to identify possible strategies which will address the experience of social isolation and loneliness, more of which is discussed later in this chapter.

The prevalence of social isolation and loneliness in the older adult

In Australia, a study found that *approximately 10% of 2000 older respondents were classified as socially isolated and another 12% were at risk of social isolation* (Gardner et al., 1998, p. 6). In an American study of over 3,000 older respondents, 35 per cent stated that they felt lonely (Anderson, 2010). In the UK, it is estimated that amongst those aged over 65, between 5 and 16 per cent report loneliness and 12 per cent feel isolated (Social Care Institute for Excellence, 2012).

Would you be surprised to learn that half a million people in the UK aged over 65 spent Christmas alone in 2009, and that, according to Age Concern, more than one in ten say they always or often feel lonely, and nearly half consider television their main form of company? More than a million people over 65 are said to feel trapped in their own home while more than 180,000 people over 65 say they have gone for a whole week without speaking to friends, neighbours or family (*Bournemouth Echo*, 2010).

It can therefore be seen that social isolation and loneliness in the older adult is a significant, and growing, public health concern in the Western world as its population ages steadily.

Now consider the following scenario.

Scenario

You are a mental health student nurse on placement with a community mental health nurse visiting Jim. Jim is a 69-year-old, recently widowed, Polish man, who has been referred to the community mental health team by his GP, who was concerned to see him looking dishevelled, quiet and withdrawn during a recent routine appointment.

It is 4.30, on a wet, windy and dark December afternoon; you are both sat in Jim's small flat. You had to climb four flights of unlit stairs to get to his front door (as the lift is out of order), bypassing some very drunk people shouting at each other accompanied by a large barking dog. You notice in the flat old newspapers lying about, uneaten food in the kitchen, an overflowing bin of incontinence pads and the television and radio on very loudly. There is no phone to be seen, only many photographs of his wife and family. Jim is unkempt, sat, legs tightly crossed in a large armchair, wearing ripped pyjamas holding his stick by his side. On the table next to him is an array of tablets and an empty beer can. As the community mental health nurse sits beside Jim, Jim grabs and holds his hand and begins to talk quickly and constantly about seemingly anything that comes into his head, crying whilst he does so.

Activity 9.6 — *Critical thinking*

What may lead you to think Jim might be feeling lonely or socially isolated?

What factors that you have read about in the previous paragraphs would you consider may contribute to Jim's experience of loneliness and isolation?

An outline answer is provided at the end of the chapter.

The above scenario will have given you some insight as to how you would possibly recognise signs of loneliness in an older person, but what does it actually feel like?

The experience of social isolation: the older person's view

The following quotes from an Age Concern (2008) report and a study by Mima Cattan (2011) convey poignantly how older people experience loneliness.

1. *This loneliness is a killer. It's worse than the fear I had of being bombed in London during the war.*
2. *I can go a whole week and not speak to anyone at all in person ... things are at their worst when you are poorly. You can't look after yourself and can't even get up for a glass of water. No one's there and no one cares if you are ill.*
3. *[When I was diagnosed with dementia] ... Acquaintances would 'pretend' not to see me if I was in their presence and people stopped inviting me to dinner or events. They assumed I had changed in ways that I hadn't, that I wasn't the same person any more and wasn't worthy of conversations.*
4. *Silence ... it's a different kind of silence when you're alone.*
5. *Being old is when you know all the answers but nobody asks you the questions.*

Activity 9.7 — ***Critical thinking***

What feelings do you think are being experienced and expressed within the quotes above?

An outline answer is provided at the end of the chapter.

A well-publicised research project entitled Social Isolation Week was run by a UK charity in the summer of 2011 (Cattan, 2011) to highlight the lived experience of social isolation for older people. Ten volunteers aged 22–50 years were confined to their own home for a week, without human contact, and only permitted to watch programmes on the TV and on the internet. To capture the full essence of their experiences, the volunteers uploaded videos and used social media daily, i.e. Twitter – but only one way, to ensure no contact with anyone else! The volunteers also completed a specially designed questionnaire to enable them to reflect at the end of their week. To enable the volunteers to understand some of the additional difficulties that an older person may experience they were also asked to wear diving gloves (to experience the limits of arthritis), vision-impairing glasses, leg weights (to experience the effect of wasting muscles), incontinence pads (to consider self-esteem and dignity issues) plus play an MP3 with white noise (to experience the effects of limited hearing) to mimic some possible effects of age.

Table 9.1 summarises the findings from the study.

All the volunteers felt they had learned a great deal about older people's experiences of being lonely; indeed, when they were asked how they would react if they had to repeat the experience over a period of a few months with only, for example, a monthly visit to a day centre and a weekly visit from someone delivering their shopping, they were adamant they would not wish to!

Emotional and behavioural responses to isolation
• Feelings of abandonment • Frustration • Anger • Fear of becoming more unwell physically or mentally, with no one to comfort or care for them • Feeling trapped and imprisoned in their house • Feelings of boredom • Loss of sense of humour (exacerbated by no one to 'joke with') • Lability of mood • Missing spontaneous contact, e.g. sending/receiving a text message and/or saying hello • Tiredness • Lethargy • Inability to concentrate • Loss of motivation

Table 9.1: Isolation week findings: the volunteers' experiences

They suggested that they would feel abandoned, as if they were in a prison, feel mentally unwell and generally be unable to cope with such a situation.

Interestingly, akin to the research literature on this subject, one day of the week seemed more lonely for the volunteers compared to the others. The volunteers felt that Friday was the worst day, similar to the research suggesting that, for housebound older people, Sunday is the worst day.

Activity 9.8 — *Reflection*

- Why do you think the young volunteers felt that Friday was the most difficult day and the one when they felt most lonely?
- Why do you think that older people may feel that Sunday is the most difficult day and the one when they felt most lonely?

As this is a reflection there is no outline answer at the end of the chapter.

When thinking about the above two questions you may have considered the weekends and the social activity implications. Fridays and Saturdays are the days of the week when younger adults are perhaps most likely to go out to socialise with friends and family, therefore in this study the volunteers would have been more aware on the Friday that they would not be seeing friends or joining in with any activities over the coming weekend. Research suggests that older adults are most likely to socialise on a Sunday, either by going out or receiving visitors, therefore they experience the same sense of loneliness when it is another Sunday spent alone.

The impacts of social isolation and social inclusion on well-being

The social environment is now recognised to be as important as genetic or biological factors on the positive or negative experience of ageing (Caccioppo, 2002). As can be seen from the above study and almost a decade of research, there are negative physical and mental health impacts that experiencing social isolation or loneliness can have on well-being.

Brownie and Horstmanhof (2011) confirm that a lack or loss of companionship and an inability to integrate into the social environment are critical correlates of loneliness and social isolation. James House (2001) entitled his editorial comment for *Psychosomatic Medicine*, 'Social isolation kills, but how and why?' This title conveys the seriousness of the impacts of social isolation and loneliness. Ong et al. (2012) state that the pain of experiencing loneliness can produce changes in the body that mimic the ageing process generally, as well as increasing the risk of heart disease (Hawkley and Caccioppo, 2010). It has been very well documented in the literature, e.g. by Cornwell and Waite (2009) and Nicholson (2012), that social isolation and loneliness negatively affect both physical and mental health, particularly among older adults (House, 2001; Tomaka et al., 2006). Indeed, the effects of social isolation and loneliness have been compared in magnitude to the damaging health effects of smoking cigarettes and other major health risks such as excessive alcohol intake, an unhealthy diet and little physical activity (House, 2001) (Table 9.2).

The impacts of social isolation and loneliness on well-being	**The positive health impacts of social involvement and inclusion**
Socially isolated people are likely to die at two to three times the rate of people with a network of social relationships and sources of emotional support (Brunner, 1997) Impacts on all-cause mortality and morbidity as well as cardiovascular disease (House, 2001) Increased risk of developing cognitive dysfunction and Alzheimer's disease (Wilson et al., 2007) Lengthened recovery rates from acute or chronic illnesses (Wilson et al., 2007) Increased risk of acquiring infections and reduced immunity (Kiecolt-Glaser et al., 1984; Pressman and Cohen, 2005) Increased risk of hospitalisation (Faulkner et al., 2003) Increased risk of falls (Mistry et al., 2001)	Enhanced social activities may help to increase the quality and length of life (Glass et al., 1999, p. 482) A higher sense of well-being and better general health (Machielse, 2006) Increased likelihood of pursuing health-enhancing behaviours, e.g. exercise, healthy eating (Kinney et al., 2005) or adhering to a beneficial medical regime Increased likelihood of reducing risky behaviours such as smoking, drinking too much, poor diet Social and productive and/or meaningful activities are as effective as fitness activities in lowering mortality (Glass et al., 1999) Maintenance of self-esteem and health and well-being generally (World Health Organization, 2007a).

The impacts of social isolation and loneliness on well-being	The positive health impacts of social involvement and inclusion
Increased risk of catching the common cold virus (Cohen et al., 1997) Increased risk of alcoholism, chronic physical health conditions, anxiety, depression, suicide and suicidal ideation, as well as poor self-rated physical health (Stanley et al., 2010) Note: Although loneliness is a key factor in depression in later life, it is worth considering whether the presence of depression and its symptoms, including withdrawal from others, in itself contributes to experiencing loneliness, the question being: which comes first? (McCrae et al., 2005, cited by Nicholson, 2012)	Increased immune function (Cohen et al., 1997; Pressman and Cohen, 2005) Increased sense of personal control over life (Cornman et al., 2003) A stronger sense of identity, role within a group and increased self-respect as social intercourse with others offers feedback to inform and develop a sense of self Personal involvement in communities and groups enhances feelings of security and sense of 'embeddedness' within society, contributing to a sense of well-being The opportunities for emotional support enhance mental well-being, as does the opportunity for practical support, e.g. as regards finances/benefits, health promotion, transport and travelling

Table 9.2: Summary of the impacts of social isolation and social exclusion

Fioto (2002) summarises thus: *Social isolation is a concept that greatly affects a person's sense of well-being and increases the risk of negative alterations in emotional and physical health* (Fioto, 2002, p. 53). Studies have shown that it is not only more common in the elderly, but that this age group typically have increased difficulty coping with its numerous effects (Fioto, 2002).

Table 9.2 highlights what the Social Care Institute for Excellence (2012) states: that tackling social isolation and loneliness is a public health and well-being issue. You, as a nurse, are involved in the promotion of your clients' health and well-being and, as Holley suggests (2007), you are in an ideal position to reduce social isolation and promote social inclusion.

Dementia, social isolation and loneliness

In the community, it is suggested that experiencing dementia may further isolate older people because of a loss of social roles: *when people cannot live up to previously held roles, or those roles are taken away from them, they are less able to contribute to their families and communities, despite their strong desire to remain involved* (Phinney, 2008). Saczynski et al. (2006) suggest that a diagnosis of dementia is clearly linked with a decreasing number of social engagements in later life. Indeed, research highlights that dementia sufferers can feel invisible (Beattie et al., 2004) as friends drift away over time or others become fearful of them when they are told the diagnosis.

Morris and Morris (2010) highlight that individuals experiencing dementia could experience a shrinking world as they may lose closeness or intimacy, lose their social world as it once was and lose sight of their future held life goals, as well as their self-identity. All of these factors can contribute to a sense of loneliness, not just for the sufferer but for the carer also, as a mutual but separate sense of detachment from the world occurs alongside their changing roles with each other, e.g. the perceived transition from husband to carer. People with dementia may also increasingly feel less familiar and comfortable with the world around them, either inside or outside their own home, reducing confidence and increasing fear leading them to withdraw into themselves and retreat from the frightening environment around them. This can be compounded by no longer being able to drive or travel comfortably and a fear of becoming lost. There is also the issue of communication; Clare (2002) reports that for those given a diagnosis of dementia there may not only be difficulty in expressing themselves but also in following conversations.

As has been alluded to earlier, with demographic and societal changes, family are often no longer the centre of the older adult's social network. Therefore as Ward et al. (2011) suggest:

> *paying attention to friendships in the lives of those with dementia [and all older people] helps to de-centre the 'family' in how we picture the support available to them, and open up our thinking to alternative sources of help and social connection in people's lives as well as to understanding the support and care that people with dementia provide to others.*
> (Ward et al., 2011, p. 4)

Living Well with Dementia (Department of Health, 2009b) sets out the UK government's strategy for helping people with dementia and their carers over the next five years. Its aim is to ensure that significant improvements are made to dementia services and the strategy has, as objective 5, to develop *peer support and learning networks* through, e.g. support groups and dementia cafes for people with dementia and their carers. The intention is to provide practical and emotional support, reduce social isolation and promote self-help. This goes some way towards addressing the loss of family support for many older people.

The importance of friendships

When considering the literature pertaining to social isolation and loneliness, it becomes evident that it is the quality of the contact that is important, not just the number of contacts. This is best expressed as a friendship. Indeed, the importance of friendships and peer support cannot be underestimated as a factor for health and well-being for the older adult. Cattan et al. (2003, 2005) confirm that family, when present in the older person's life, may not be in fact a source of emotional support, even though adult children may offer practical support.

Activity 9.9 **Reflection**

- How many friends would you say you had in your life right now?
- What roles do friends play in your life? Do these roles vary depending on who the friend is, e.g. a close friend or not?
- How do your friends make you feel about yourself and your life?

As this is a reflection there is no outline answer at the end of the chapter.

Routsalo et al. (2009) suggest that groups of older people who meet weekly are useful ways of increasing the size of social networks and number of friends, thus increasing well-being, with Cattan et al. (2005) highlighting that the inclusion of educational (talks) and social activities (cards and games) within these groups is a key factor.

Research summary: the importance of friendship

A study undertaken by a university in the south of England with a local charity explored the impact of older people attending weekly friendship clubs (run similarly to those described in the paragraph above), addressing social isolation and loneliness (Jack, 2011). The research found that older people recognised having friendships as helping prevent loneliness and social isolation in many ways.

(a) The older people felt that by simply having and mixing with friends, their core identity and sense of who they are were reinforced, e.g. by remembering and celebrating significant events, joyful (birthdays) or otherwise (bereavements).

(b) They liked being able to gossip confidentially with friends and peers from the same age group; indeed, being in the company of friends enabled them to talk about anything without fear of repercussions or being judged.

(c) These friendships with others of a similar age, interests, experiences, personal history and historical background ensured mutual benefit for all involved, e.g. the sharing of life experiences (good and bad) as well as allowing the sharing of a particular worldview that was felt to come only with age. Being able to help and support others was deemed as essential for well-being. The sharing of jokes was also seen as very important!

(d) The weekly opportunity for meeting with and making friends provided company/companionship, as the actual presence of someone (as opposed to the television) for conversation was important. True friendship was depicted as *being seen as an equal, an individual and being treated with respect and dignity* by others, whereby they felt listened to and never made to feel boring!

(e) The companionship was especially important for those who had lost a partner. They described the clubs as providing the opportunity to recapture the activities previously enjoyed with a partner, e.g. watching/discussing a sunset, or a trip out, or even simply talking about the newspapers or TV, plus there was also the opportunity for significant emotional/romantic relationships.

(f) A crucial finding from this study was that the older people described their ability to address loneliness themselves, by turning up at the clubs and making the best of the opportunity offered to them to build, sustain or make new friendships that extended activities beyond the club itself, e.g. attending local events together, or perhaps simply meeting for coffee/lunch or even just making regular telephone calls to each other where mobility or travelling was an issue.

Activity 9.10 *The older person's view of friendships*

Here are some comments made by the older people in the study. Can you match what they said to the points in the research summary?

1. We all have our growing up in common – or similar.
2. We understand when we talk to each other and have a laugh about our aches and pains because we've got it too!
3. Friends listen and have time for you … they would never let you think that you are boring.
4. You can talk about anything and they wouldn't disrespect you.
5. Before, I would walk into town and not know anybody … now I will walk into town and see people from the club even just to say hello to, which is nice.
6. Seeing a face you recognise at church from the club … it's so nice.
7. It's lovely to go on the trips out with friends, I missed that when my husband died, just being somewhere different and having something else to talk about makes a difference.
8. It's important you know, to feel like you have something to offer – sometimes it's sympathy, sometimes it's advice for my friends … it's good to feel useful and valued – like the person I used to be.
9. My friends are always pleased to see me – that makes me feel like a person … who I am … not just that old biddy in the mirror.
10. I feel like my, old, well young self again!

An outline answer is provided at the end of the chapter.

Having done the last activity, do you notice any similarities between what the older people in the study felt about the value of friendships, and what you noted for yourself in the reflective Activity 9.9? The next activity will help you identify some of the similarities.

Activity 9.11 *Reflection*

Thinking back to the reflective Activity 9.9, in particular consider the following two questions again for yourself and your own friends, and compare them to what you have just read about older people and the value of friendships.

- What roles do friends play in your life? Do these roles vary depending on who the friend is, e.g. a close friend or not?
- How do your friends make you feel about yourself and your life?

You may notice that your thoughts about the value of your own friendships mirror those of the older people in the study!

As this is a reflection there is no outline answer at the end of the chapter.

Consider the following light-hearted short article by David Newnham which seems to sum up the value of friendships as one grows older.

Case study: David Newnham, in 2012

It might come as a surprise to anyone under 50, but getting older can actually be fun. Whoever would have thought it? ... I mean the fun to be had sharing the common experience of ageing. A bit like what Australians call 'moan bonding', only more upbeat. More fun, in fact. Take Rick and I. He took early retirement two years ago and I ran into him at the weekend. Was he missing work? I had to be joking. Was he making ends meet? Not so you would notice. And how was his health? A quarter past two. A quarter past what? Oh, right. It was a joke about his hearing. 'I thought it was wax, but the doc said it is basically my age.' Me too, I said. 'Quarter past,' he replied. After hearing loss, it was blood pressure. The two of us compared medication like a couple of kids swapping football cards. Did he have the diuretics? Did he have the ones that give you a cough? Did he ever forget to take them? We both had dodgy discs, peered through varifocals and swallowed statins. But the greatest source of hilarity was the senior moments – the missing names, lost threads and words that vanish without trace. We both realise these things will only get worse, but knowing we are in the same boat means we can relish the absurdity of it all. Can you imagine teenagers comparing notes about adolescence? Ugh. Embarrassing. But life is too short for embarrassment and the more I see of this ageing malarkey, the more convinced I am that someone up there is having a laugh with us. And there is nothing I enjoy more than a good laugh.
(Newnham, 2012, p. 25)

Addressing loneliness and social isolation: what you can do

We will focus in this chapter on the home and community setting as many of the interventions and principles are the same.

As we have seen throughout this chapter, social isolation and loneliness can be detrimental to an older person's health, well-being and quality of life. The World Health Organization (2007a) suggests that participation in leisure, social, cultural and spiritual activities, for example, in the community, helps older people maintain self-esteem, maintain or create supportive and caring relationships by fostering social integration and is the key to staying informed. There is a need for all sectors (health, social care, voluntary, charity) to work together in providing interventions to address this with a key focus on recognising that they should be asset-based interventions. As the research above identified, older people do have the skills and capacity to take ownership of these interventions which will also instil a sense of self-empowerment, crucial for well-being. This is important to note as it highlights the empowering and enabling approach you as a nurse can take.

We know that older people are not a homogeneous group. We need to adopt a humanised, person-centred approach (recognising that the older person is the expert on his or her experiences, view of life and well-being). You as a nurse now know that loneliness/social isolation is what people experience and describe for themselves: it is a perceived lack of meaningful contact with others, regardless of how socially isolated or not they may be. This also sits well with the humanising framework mentioned in Chapter 1 (Todres et al., 2009), which recognises the individuality of people on their unique journey through life and crucially their need to be in relationships and thus connected with others.

Interventions over the last few years that have been used to tackle social isolation or loneliness include befriending, mentoring and social group schemes. There have been many reviews of the research literature as to the nature of interventions such as these but there is little consensus as to what actually works for older people.

What can I do as nurse to encourage social inclusion with the older person?

In a professional role

As stated earlier, Holley (2007) suggests that nurses are in an ideal position to reduce social isolation and promote social inclusion. In doing so, however, it is important that, as a nurse, you recognise that older people have assets and skills. Therefore engaging in the therapeutic relationship and with sensitive assessment, you can establish clients' desires for social involvement and harness their abilities and skills to address this. For example, do they think they would benefit from considering widening their social networks and number of friends? Remember that older people are often reluctant to admit to feeling lonely or isolated, so tackling this subject needs a great deal of sensitivity.

What can you suggest to enhance the well-being of the older person with regard to reducing social isolation and loneliness? Whether in the hospital, residential or community setting, it is always useful to find out for yourself first what is available in the local area for older people to do and become involved in – think about what you might like to be doing when you are older, or what an older relative of yours might wish to do and seek out information from there.

As we know, lack of transport and fear of travelling on public transport can be significant barriers for older people when considering engaging with others. Many activities/organisations provide transport and/or escorting. This is always important to know about before sharing your suggestions with older people, as they may be very disappointed to find out about an ideal activity only to find that they cannot get there! Be mindful also of cost implications for some activities; do not suggest activities to the older person if they are costly and you are aware that the person has financial limitations.

Information and signposting services for clients can be very useful as accessing these involves the client in having to make the contact and thus take control, e.g. Partnerships for Older People Projects/Wayfinder/Community Navigators (see useful websites, below, for further details as to what these services offer). These services guide clients to access services that may help them practically, including health and social services and assessments, plus offer charity and volunteer activities to participate in.

In terms of individual support, if you sense or assess that older clients may be feeling isolated or lonely, you may wish to encourage them to take action in activities that reflect their interests, e.g. what activities does the local theatre, cinema, history group or library offer? You could also contact the local religious organisation, e.g. church, mosque or a local charity for information on activities available, e.g. Age Concern. Their GP practice may know of locally based services offered by the health or social care sector, e.g. day centre services often provide lunch clubs and focused activity groups such as reading or creative writing.

Health promotion activities can also be useful in addressing social isolation for the older adult. Most areas offer fitness classes for people over 50 in local leisure centres and many further education centres offer classes and advice on, for example, nutrition and healthy ageing.

Befriending/mentoring, buddying and partnering schemes not only help to provide much-needed company but can also practically assist in getting out and about and (re-)engaging in activities such as those described above. Some organisations, e.g. Contact, organise for older people to meet over tea and cake.

Wider community engagement projects can enable older people to become involved in volunteering activities, thus making use of their knowledge and skills, e.g. local volunteer centres of Time Banks (see useful websites at the end of the chapter).

Where the use of technology (computers and the internet for chat forums of shared interest) is not an option, perhaps a letter-writing or penpal forum could be useful, e.g. as provided through Amnesty International. If the older person does not have access to a useful telephone, e.g. due to hearing/sight loss, again the health/social care sector or charities can be involved in obtaining and assisting with the costs of these.

It may even be a possibility for the older person to become a pet owner as there is research that indicates that having an animal companion is a very effective strategy in overcoming loneliness. Support from other services may be required to support the older person with this; some veterinary surgeries offer free services to support older people in keeping their animal companions healthy and local authority services can often assist also, e.g. volunteer dog walkers.

Joining educational activities such as courses or book clubs can be suggested, perhaps through organisations such as the University of the Third Age. Indeed, older people may even be able to take part in teaching the courses! You may feel that specialist groups may be of use for social support at a particular time, e.g. during bereavement (Cruse), or a recent diagnosis of a physical condition, e.g. the Stroke Association.

It may be that you consider with clients whether their current living arrangements are contributing. Do they need to consider moving to a warden-controlled environment, or a community arrangement such as a residential/nursing home in order to alleviate their feelings of isolation?

In summary, as a nurse you must have knowledge and awareness of the services and agencies that can prevent or alleviate loneliness in older age, either to offer supporting individual strategies or involvement in group activities/interventions, which may be social, cultural or even health-promoting in nature.

In a personal capacity

The Isolation Week study mentioned earlier suggests the following six things you can do personally:

1. If you see an older person struggling, for example in the supermarket, ask if you can help – and then stop to have a chat if the person wants.
2. Don't forget your own older relatives and friends – try to call or visit them. Stay in touch.
3. Remember older people's birthdays – send them a card.
4. Regularly check on older neighbours or friends – drop by for a chat.
5. Become a volunteer – either with Friends of the Elderly (**www.fote.org.uk**) or find other volunteering opportunities at **www.do-it.org**.
6. Support Friends of the Elderly to provide more services – donate at **http://www.fote.org.uk/support-us/donate**.

Most importantly, remember and recognise older people as, and as having, assets. They have a lifetime of knowledge and experience with the skills to match. Ensure your own attitudes and behaviour reflect this understanding in your actions and challenge others who do not, and demonstrate ageist, discriminatory and stigmatising values.

Consider the following quote to remind yourself of what older people may already have residing within themselves.

> *Happiness is being 74 – The young have stress, ambition, unfulfilled dreams. The elderly have contentment.*
> (Bakewell, J (2010) *The Guardian*, Tuesday 23 February)

Scenario

You are out on a visit with a community physiotherapist and occupational therapist to visit Mrs Courson, a 74-year-old woman who has recently been discharged home from a medical ward at a local hospital after a small stroke which left her with little use of her left arm and limited mobility. She has, up until now, lived alone, and very independently since her husband died five years ago. Mrs Courson has one daughter who now lives in Australia and, although they have frequent telephone contact, they have not seen each other for many years. Before being admitted to hospital Mrs Courson had an active social life with

(continued)

continued ...

many friends, going out every day either shopping or attending her many social engagements and volunteering activities (clubs and events with friends), either driving or travelling by public transport. She has limited finances, living off her pension.

During the assessment process, supporting aids and some house modifications were suggested to Mrs Courson, who agreed to them all, as well as accepting that she was unable to drive for the time being. Her main concern however was worry about being able to go out as she now felt anxious and afraid of falling or even having another stroke. You and the occupational therapist then discuss how Mrs Courson can best be supported to recover and maintain her health, well-being and quality of life.

Activity 9.12 — *Critical thinking*

Read the scenario, and then answer the following questions:

What factors can you identify that may suggest Mrs Courson could be at risk of becoming isolated or lonely?

What topics might you and the occupational therapist wish to discuss with Mrs Courson when considering promoting her health and well-being?

When trying to answer these questions, think about what you are basing your answers on.

An outline answer is provided at the end of the chapter.

Dickens et al. (2011) suggest from long-term studies that group interventions eg. where groups are set up for older people to come together, may be more beneficial than 1:1 interventions, e.g. one person going to visit the lonely individual in their home or vice versa. These group interventions are also best when they have a social focus offering opportunities for emotional and practical support. Older people described the benefits such as increasing their social interactions and connections with others and feeling part of their community again, as well as being prompted to pursue enjoyable activities, e.g. taking up or going back to hobbies. These group interventions sit well with the research study mentioned earlier which had friendship as a focus.

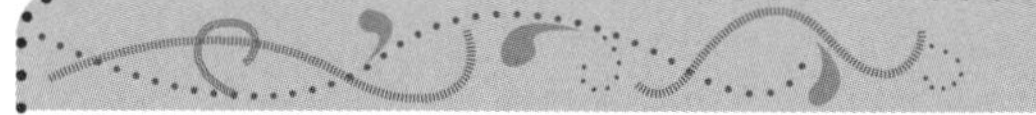

Chapter summary

This chapter has explored the meaning and experience of social isolation and loneliness in current society for the older person and the negative impacts that these experiences can have on health and well-being. It has highlighted that it can be addressed through harnessing and empowering older people's ability to establish and maintain meaningful social relationships and friendships, thus empowering them as individuals. Importantly, the strong positive relationship between friendship and well-being (Larson, 1978; Wood and Robertson, 1978) has been clearly articulated. The chapter has identified the role that the nurse in her professional role (and personal life) can have as a facilitator and enabler in working with older people reflecting the paradigm shift highlighting the move from a 'needs-led' approach to an 'assets-led' approach in working with clients.

Activities: brief outline answers

Activity 9.2

The social worker may have made his or her own assessment as to the actual number of people that the client had contact with on a regular basis, that is, that the client had few, if any, social contacts, neither friends nor family, to share his everyday life with.

The volunteer may have noticed that the older person seemed withdrawn, saying that he had not spoken to anyone since his last visit, nor had he been out of his house, and that he missed the company of his wife and family more than ever since his wife died and his family moved abroad.

Activity 9.3

Einstein was suggesting that being alone in later life can often be very enjoyable after a busy life in previous years, a chance to be on one's own without interruption and enjoy one's own company. Often, during very busy times in life, it can be healthy to stop, and be by ourself. This gives us time to reflect and take stock of where we are and where we are going in life. It can give us the opportunity to see solutions to challenges as well as appreciating the good things in our lives. It also gives us the chance to pursue those solo activities that make us happy. It could be suggested that it is always more enjoyable, however, when that solitude is chosen, not enforced upon us.

Holley intimates this by saying that *A person's choice to seek solitude at times is healthy. Solitude is voluntarily chosen time alone for reflecting, centering, feeling spiritually connected, and finding inner peace and strength* (Holley, 2007, p. 51).

Activity 9.6

Feeling lonely Jim has not been going out to buy newspapers recently or dispose of his rubbish. No one has been in to see him to offer/give help. The radio and television may be his only form of company. There is no working telephone for him to contact others. He is not dressed and is not taking care of his appearance, therefore perhaps not expecting anyone to visit and with no plans to go out. He grabs the nurse – needing to touch another human being? Is Jim missing his wife and family – are they in Poland?

Contributing factors Mobility issues – frailty, difficulty managing the stairs which are also unlit and fears for safety regarding others and their behaviour, especially during inclement weather and darkness.

Is incontinence an issue – or is his general physical health (medication side-effects?) impacting on his willingness and confidence to go out?

Is Jim depressed following his bereavement – not eating and self-caring?

Does he find communication difficult – in terms of language or culture?

Activity 9.7

Within the first quote, you may consider that there is a strong sense of fear, a fear of dying alone, indeed perhaps from the loneliness itself. Within quote two, again you may note that fear is present, the fear of being ill and alone, unable to take care of oneself and therefore feeling helpless. Perhaps you may think there is also a sense of disappointment and anger at being let down by friends/family or indeed society, that the person should be so alone and uncared for in later life. Within quote three, you may note that there is a suggestion of stigma attached to the diagnosis of dementia, being excluded as others no longer acknowledge the person they once were, as if their (self) identity disintegrated when the diagnosis was shared. Perhaps a loss of role was experienced, that of friend alongside an overall loss of dignity and personhood. The fourth quote perhaps highlights the lack of choice an older person has with regard to choosing solitude or not; in this case solitude seems to be imposed rather than chosen. The final quote perhaps highlights the feelings of being subject to ageism, discrimination or stigma from society as, despite the fact the older person recognises her wisdom, she feels that no one wishes to ask her for an opinion, she has no voice and even if she did, no one would value hearing it.

Activity 9.10

Depending on your interpretation and understanding of what was said, the answers may vary. However as a suggested answer please refer to the table below.

Comment	Point in list
9, 1	(a)
1, 4, 10	(b)
8, 2, 1	(c)
3	(d)
7	(e)
6, 5	(f)

Activity 9.12

Below is only a brief outline of what may be discussed and suggested.

First of all you must be sensitive to the fact that Mrs Courson may not wish to disclose that she feels at risk of becoming lonely and discuss the topic gently.

You may have considered the fact that Mrs Courson is feeling anxious and nervous about her health generally, suggesting a loss of confidence in her abilities and also perhaps a loss of her concept of self as she is currently faced daily with evidence of her compromised health (limited mobility and limited use of left arm) and the possibility of not being able to carry on those everyday activities that she finds enjoyable due to being unable to drive and nervous of travelling on public transport. Her ability to self-care in personal hygiene and dress independently (wearing the clothes and accessories that she would usually wear) may also impact on her identity and self-esteem and cause reluctance to meet with others due to embarrassment. She may feel her self-esteem falling as she cannot volunteer for the time being, thus offering support to others, and she may also be concerned that she would have nothing interesting to say or talk about if she did meet with other people, whether she went out to visit them or they came to visit her.

You may wish to talk to Mrs Courson about what usually makes her happy in her life. What fulfils, inspires and motivates her on a daily basis? What does she usually enjoy doing? In this way you can establish with her what she needs to do to maintain and enhance her well-being. You can then establish with her ways in which these activities can be preserved. Could any of her friends accompany her on public transport? Could they provide a lift in a car, or perhaps visit regularly? Local volunteer or charity organisations may also be able to provide both those services at little or no cost.

The occupational therapist may wish to suggest some work to enhance her self-esteem, e.g. bibliotherapy, psychoeducation, or consider a referral to the mental health services for a brief intervention to screen/ address possible depressive symptoms. The occupational therapist could also review Mrs Courson's current skills pertaining to her ability to dress herself as she would wish and supply aids and suggestions/modifications to ensure she can still dress as she wishes or receive daily care until such time as she can attend to herself independently.

There may be a volunteer befriending scheme locally that could help by visiting or telephoning. Ideally, however, it is best to ensure Mrs Courson attends her usual activities and meets groups of others outside the home, so there could be discussion as to whether there are any voluntary car-driving services locally that may be able to take her to and from her usual activities. There may be Stroke Association self-help groups in the area that she could attend for support with her condition and to share her experiences for others or a stroke-specific Wayfinders/Community Navigator volunteer programme. This type of programme seeks to give people the knowledge of the available services and talks them through the process, so they are empowered to make the transition from being managed by their condition to managing it. Go to: **http://www.institute.nhs.uk/hsca/national/_content/health_and_social_care_-_past_winners/national_winners_and_finalists_2006/community_care_navigators.aspx**.

Useful websites

http://www.rcn.org.uk/development/practice/social_inclusion/social_inclusion_uk_agenda/policy

This is the Royal College of Nursing webpage which has a focus on social inclusion.

http://www.scie.org.uk

This is an excellent web resource from the Social Care Institute for Excellence, which is an independent charity working with adults, families and children's social care and social work services across the UK.

http://www.contact-the-elderly.org.uk

This website is from Contact the Elderly, the only national charity solely dedicated to tackling loneliness and social isolation among older people.

http://www.fote.org.uk

This charity offers a wide variety of services, including residential care homes, nursing care homes and dementia care homes, as well as day clubs and befriending schemes.

The Friends of the Elderly organisation has a further isolation information link to follow, highlighting the research exploring social isolation:

http://www.fote.org.uk/wp-content/uploads/2012/11/Sources-for-Infographic-FINAL.pdf

http://campaigntoendloneliness.org/toolkit/wp-content/uploads/Services-to-reduce-loneliness-and-isolation-amongst-older-people.pdf

The above link provides a list of suggestions for health and well-being boards to reduce loneliness and social isolation.

http://www.thesilverline.org.uk

This is the website for a telephone initiative to tackle loneliness that offers both telephone befriending as well as practical information and advice – a national helpline for elderly people which they can call for assistance with anything that is troubling them. It is funded by the Comic Relief charity, with other organisations, e.g. BT, offering its services for free.

www.supportline.org.uk

This is a support line for people who feel socially isolated.

www.ageuk.org.uk/professional-resources-home/knowledge-hub-evidence-statistics/research-community/social-inclusion-and-loneliness-research

This website provides links to academic research units, funders and charities that focus on addressing social inclusion and loneliness in the older person.

www.do-it.org.uk

This website has general information related to volunteering.

http://timebank.org.uk

The Time Bank facilitates formal and informal volunteering activities through established projects and miscellaneous community events.

Chapter 10
Interprofessional collaboration when working with older people

Sarah Hean and Sue Smith

NMC Standards for Pre-registration Nursing Education

Domain 1: Communication and interpersonal skills

1. All nurses must build partnerships and therapeutic relationships through safe, effective and non-discriminatory communication. They must take account of individual differences, capabilities and needs.
2. All nurses must use a range of communication skills and technologies to support person-centred care and enhance quality and safety. They must ensure people receive all the information they need in a language and manner that allows them to make informed choices and share decision making. They must recognise when language interpretation or other communication support is needed and know how to obtain it.
3. Nurses must use the full range of communication methods, including verbal, non-verbal and written, to acquire, interpret and record their knowledge and understanding of people's needs. They must be aware of their own values and beliefs and the impact this may have on their communication with others. They must take account of the many different ways in which people communicate and how these may be influenced by ill health, disability and other factors, and be able to recognise and respond effectively when a person finds it hard to communicate.
4. All nurses must recognise when people are anxious or in distress and respond effectively, using therapeutic principles, to promote their wellbeing, manage personal safety and resolve conflict. They must use effective communication strategies and negotiation techniques to achieve best outcomes, respecting the dignity and human rights of all concerned. They must know when to consult a third party and how to make referrals for advocacy, mediation or arbitration.

Domain 3: Nursing practice and decision making

1. All nurses must use up-to-date knowledge and evidence to assess, plan, deliver and evaluate care, communicate findings, influence change and promote health and best

(continued)

continued ...

practice. They must make person-centred, evidence-based judgments and decisions, in partnership with others involved in the care process, to ensure high quality care. They must be able to recognise when the complexity of clinical decisions requires specialist knowledge and expertise, and consult or refer accordingly.

10. All nurses must evaluate their care to improve clinical decision-making, quality and outcomes, using a range of methods, amending the plan of care, where necessary, and communicating changes to others.

Domain 4: Leadership, management and team working

7. All nurses must use up-to-date knowledge and evidence to assess, plan, deliver and evaluate care, communicate findings, influence change and promote health and best practice. They must make person-centred, evidence-based judgments and decisions, in partnership with others involved in the care process, to ensure high quality care. They must be able to recognise when the complexity of clinical decisions requires specialist knowledge and expertise, and consult or refer accordingly.

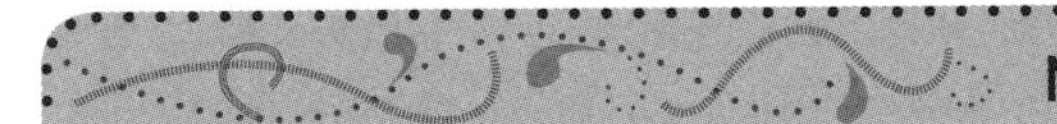

NMC Essential Skills Clusters (ESCs)

This chapter will support the following ESCs:

Care, compassion and communication

1. As partners in the care process, people can trust a newly registered graduate nurse to provide collaborative care based on the highest standards, knowledge and competence.
4. People can trust a newly qualified graduate nurse to engage with them and their family or carers within their cultural environments in an acceptant and anti-discriminatory manner free from harassment and exploitation.
6. People can trust the newly registered graduate nurse to engage therapeutically and actively listen to their needs and concerns, responding using skills that are helpful, providing information that is clear, accurate, meaningful and free from jargon.

Organisational aspects of care

14. People can trust the newly registered graduate nurse to be an autonomous and confident member of the multi-disciplinary or multi-agency team and to inspire confidence in others.
15. People can trust the newly registered graduate nurse to safely delegate to others and to respond appropriately when a task is delegated to them.
19. People can trust the newly registered graduate nurse to work to prevent and resolve conflict and maintain a safe environment.

Chapter aims

By the end of this chapter, you will be able to:

- define interprofessional collaborative practice accurately;
- develop strategies to communicate with other professional groups and the older patient in a collaborative and respectful manner;
- demonstrate an awareness of the importance of being able to articulate your own professional role and that of other professional groups when caring for an older person;
- engage the older person as a central member of the interprofessional team;
- recognise that conflict is a normal part of interprofessional working and be able to develop strategies to resolve this;
- understand and apply some key principles of interprofessional leadership;
- understand some of the principles of team functioning that enable effective interprofessional collaboration.

Introduction

Mary has just retired. She and her husband live in a small village on the south coast of England. Mary's mother, Charlotte, is 85 years of age and lives alone in a bungalow a few miles from Mary, her husband having died six years ago. Charlotte is not in good health. She has angina and diabetes, is hard of hearing, having suffered with mastoids as a child, and has a severe prolapse, which is inoperable because of her general health. We will meet Charlotte and Mary again in this chapter.

As people get older, the likelihood of developing multiple and longer-term needs increases. Collaboration between a wide range of professionals and organisations is required to address these. An ageing population in many Western countries means that a large number of patients will be older (Soule et al., 2005) and the need for collaboration between professionals will become increasingly important. Health and social care professionals must therefore develop the knowledge and skills required to collaborate effectively at an interagency and interprofessional level.

This chapter explains the meaning of interprofessional collaboration and its benefits to older people. It then describes the key interprofessional collaborative competencies healthcare professionals must develop if they are to care effectively for this population group.

Benefits of interprofessional working

The way in which health and social care is delivered has become increasingly dependent on team and interagency working and it is reassuring that evidence suggests that interprofessional team working does improve patient/client outcomes. Shapiro et al. (2001), for example, in a study of healthcare teams, concluded that the more people who are members of an interprofessional team, the better the outcomes for the patient. This may be because the mix of skills and knowledge that each member brings to the team increases innovation and creativity. Similarly, in a systematic review of interprofessional working around older people in the community, Trivedi et al. (2012) found that interagency partnerships that had some mechanism for different professionals to work together and shared assessment procedures and records between different agencies reduced the levels of hospital and nursing home use.

What does interprofessional collaborative practice mean?

The World Health Organization defines interprofessional collaborative practice as occurring when *multiple health workers from different professional backgrounds provide comprehensive services by working with patients, their families, carers and communities to deliver the highest quality of care across settings* (World Health Organization, 2010a, p. 13).

Collaboration can occur between different professionals within one organisation or increasingly between professionals who belong to a range of organisations from the public, private and third sectors. Collaboration is not necessarily only required between health workers. Social workers, police, lawyers, teachers, probation officers and charity workers, for example, are part of the wider interprofessional team supporting an older person's needs. In this chapter the case studies follow Charlotte, who receives care both in the community and later in hospital.

Case study part 1: Charlotte at home

Charlotte and her late husband had had a traditional relationship. Charlotte had stayed at home to care for Mary and her brother, while Mary's father had gone out to work and taken responsibility for the family finances. Mary describes her relationship with Charlotte as being far from a good mother–daughter one and describes a level of resentment, having recently retired from a busy job, and that her mother now expects her to drop everything to be her full-time carer. Mary describes feeling guilty about feeling this way but sees her experience as Charlotte's main carer as one of frustration.

About six months ago, Mary began to worry more about Charlotte, noticing she had stopped washing herself. Mary is concerned that her mother no longer cares what she looks like. She wishes she would take pride in her personal appearance again and in her bungalow. Mary is concerned that her mother appears to have given up on herself and may be lonely.

Mary describes herself as a good organiser and has become a key coordinator of Charlotte's care. She had a sit-in shower fitted for Charlotte that has worked well. She realised her mother is not able physically to clean the bungalow any more, so she managed to get Charlotte to agree to a cleaner for two hours a week and a gardener for two hours every fortnight.

Mary has researched the benefits available to her mother, and found out that Charlotte is entitled to the high rate of attendance allowance, although she has difficulty persuading Charlotte to claim this money.

Mary has contacted numerous agencies to support Charlotte, including Age UK, social services, the local GP surgery and local church groups. She has experience of doing this from looking for support for her adult son who has learning difficulties.

All the agencies she has approached have been very helpful. They have summed up Charlotte's needs and looked into Mary's needs also. They have carried out assessments offering suggestions for how Charlotte can get out and about, what care she needs and general helpful information. Mary describes the various professionals as having always had a caring, listening ear and been sympathetic to what she is saying but comments that sometimes they do not see the full picture: 'They see my mother as an archetypal old lady with silver hair in a bun and a willing smile. If only they knew', says Mary.

Sometimes Charlotte appears not to cooperate. She insists, when meeting with agency representatives, that she does not need help, and does not get lonely or depressed. She has rejected the offer of a 'befriending' service offered by one of the local age charities but privately admits to Mary that she is very down.

Activity 10.1 — *Critical thinking*

Read through the case study of Charlotte part 1 and consider the following questions.

- Can you identify the agencies involved in supporting Charlotte, the professionals who might work within these and the sectors they represent?
- What role does Mary play in the care of her mother?

An outline answer is provided at the end of the chapter.

From the case study you can see that Charlotte has a number of physical conditions (e.g. angina and diabetes). She is also lonely and is showing early signs of depression. Health professionals, social workers and third-sector organisations are required to provide support to improve her physical and mental well-being and practical day-to-day living. The publication of the National Service Framework for Older People (Department of Health, 2001a) recognised this need for multiple agency involvement in the care of an older person and the provision of coordinated care across this range of services. It encourages better collaborative practice across organisational and professional boundaries.

Mary talks of the number of public and third-sector organsations that she has contacted and who have assessed her mother, and for whom a level of integration is required to ensure that professionals work collaboratively together to maximise Charlotte's well-being. However, interprofessional and interagency working is not always optimal, and there are several well-known quoted incidences where failures in collaborative practices have led to serious errors in care (e.g. the death of Victoria Climbie and the public inquiry into children's heart surgery at the Bristol Royal Infirmary: Kennedy, 2001; Laming, 2003, 2009). Although nothing as serious has happened to Mary and her mother, they are aware of the frustration that a lack of collaboration between professional groups aand services can cause.

Case study part 2: Mary's experience of coordinated services in the community

Mary reports that the care of her mother and the services provided have been excellent. There has always been support for her and for Charlotte, with suggestions as to the way forward. However, communication between the agencies could have been better. She believes they would have worked better if they were able to network better and give more support to one another. On several occasions, appointments have been confused because one service had not liaised with another. Mary also reported some contradictions in the diagnosis of her mother's prolapse that had confused Charlotte unnecessarily, especially as she often had to repeat the same information over and over to different people. 'Don't they have any shared records about who's seen my mother, when and what the outcome has been?' asks Mary.

Mary also recalls an earlier event talking to the GP when Charlotte had a fall, cutting her back badly. The GP prescribes an antiseptic cream. Mary attended the consultation and was able to point out that her mother would not able to administer the cream herself in her physical condition. At Mary's insistence the GP refers to a district nurse to attend.

Activity 10.2 — *Critical thinking*

- What examples of poor communication can you observe in case study part 2?
- What could have happened to Charlotte as a result of this poor communication?

An outline answer is provided at the end of the chapter.

As a nurse you will need to work collaboratively with the patient and her family, with other professional groups and across organisational boundaries if you are to provide good care for the older person and avoid serious errors. In the rest of the chapter, we explore a range of interprofessional competencies that you should develop.

Interprofessional competencies

Interprofessional competencies are the skills and knowledge required by nurses if they are to collaborate effectively with other professionals, with a range of organisations and with different patient groups. Being non-clinical skills, these competencies can be more difficult to articulate, but Orchard and Bainbridge (2010) present us with clear guidance on the characteristics and means of operationalising six interprofessional competency domains.

These relate to:

1. interprofessional communication;
2. patient-centred care;
3. interprofessional role clarification;
4. interprofessional conflict resolution;
5. interprofessional collaborative leadership;
6. interprofessional team functioning.

We will explore each of these competencies in relation to our case study to illustrate where these competencies have or have not been demonstrated and how these might be developed by the healthcare professional involved.

Interprofessional communication

Workers from different professions should be able to communicate with each other in a collaborative, responsive and responsible manner (Orchard and Bainbridge, 2010).

Case study part 3: Charlotte in hospital

A few months later, Charlotte was admitted to hospital with a severe cough and, following examination, she was diagnosed with advanced, aggressive lung cancer. She was scared and lonely. She told staff that, whatever the diagnosis, she did not want any treatment or resuscitation, but would accept pain management.

Shortly after Charlotte was admitted, Mary and her husband, James, visited her in hospital. A young nurse greeted them warmly. She asked them about how Charlotte was feeling and if she was coming to terms with her diagnosis. Mary and James were taken aback, not having been aware of Charlotte's recent diagnosis. The nurse looked nervous, halted her conversation and excused herself rapidly. James and Mary were left alone, shocked and upset about the unexpected news.

Case study part 3 describes a breakdown of communication between the oncologist and the ward nurse on whether the family should be told or has been told of Charlotte's diagnosis. There needed to be consultation between these two professionals before the family visited.

Imagine how different James and Mary's experience might have been if time had been ring-fenced for formal and regular briefing and debriefing sessions between nursing and medical staff to improve team communication. Hereby, each professional could have volunteered and requested information on Charlotte's situation. This should be a two-way exchange of information between professional groups. The medical staff might have described Charlotte's diagnosis and the nursing staff could have provided a more holistic picture of Charlotte's family circumstances and general well-being. At such a meeting, the nurse could have volunteered that Charlotte's family was involved in her care. This might have prompted the oncologist to inform the nurse that James and Mary had not yet been informed of the diagnosis. Briefing sessions should be facilitated in such a way that all staff members have the confidence to voice their concerns or queries. If this had happened, the nurse might have been able to break the news more gently to James and Mary and have been better able to support them in coming to terms with Charlotte's diagnosis.

An essential skill within the domain of interprofessional communication is the ability to listen to other team members actively. If you are nursing in a setting where such meetings are not regularly held, you must make a conscious effort to engage with the oncologist actively, both listening to the information other professionals are providing as well as actively delivering information to them on the patient's condition. The oncologist may well have shared with her colleagues the information that Charlotte's family had not been informed, but the nurse in this case study may not have registered this in the rush of handover or during particularly busy times on the ward. Professionals should therefore make a conscious effort to listen actively as well as talk to other professional groups, understanding that others may have different priorities and ways of expressing themselves. Each profession should consciously strive towards communicating with each other in language that is free from jargon and acronyms. This ensures that all members of the team share a common understanding of care decisions.

You should also pay particular attention to actively listening to the patient. For older people, this may mean speaking extra clearly, if necessary louder and more slowly. Charlotte would have been able to inform staff, if they had actively listened to her, whether her family knew of her diagnosis and indeed if she wished them to know.

Active listening may be hindered by prejudice. Unfortunately, ageist prejudice (Department of Health, 2001a; World Health Organization, 2004, 2007a) and discrimination against older people (Liu et al., 2012) prevent healthcare professionals from active listening and lead to misunderstandings such as that described in this case study. Stereotypes are not always extreme. In case study part 1, professionals characterised Charlotte as a nice grey-haired old lady. This stereotype may have prevented them from seeing her true needs and loneliness, known only to Mary. As a nurse you should re-examine your own attitudes and prejudices towards older patients and make an effort to listen to them actively. Had the nurse actively listened to Charlotte or her family (case study part 3), she might have picked up cues earlier that the family did not know the diagnosis and have taken the time to break this to them more gently and with Charlotte's consent. By taking the time to listen actively to other professionals within the team, as well as to the older patient and family, nurses are able to build mutual trust and empathy between themselves and these other groups. Building these sorts of relationships will facilitate better team functioning and patient outcomes (Adamson, 2011).

All our interactions with patients and other health and social care workers involve non-verbal as well as verbal communication. Resentment or prejudice towards particular patient or professional groups is hard to disguise. If you harbour such feelings, reflect on why you feel this way and think of strategies to overcome them. Building trust with the older patient and other professional groups is important, as is practising the skills of listening, negotiating, consulting, interacting, discussing or debating. This takes time but, as with all skills, the more you practise, the better you become.

Mutual respect and trust also build through consistently sharing information in a way that promotes full disclosure and transparency during interactions with other team members. If nurses lack the confidence to speak up in an interprofessional case conference, for example, they may inadvertently not disclose the indepth knowledge they have of the patient's personal circumstances with the rest of the team, leading to poor patient outcomes (Reid, 2012). Imagine you are a newly appointed ward nurse, and you have noticed that the family of a patient has not been informed of a patient's diagnosis but no one appears to have taken responsibility for informing them of this or consulting the patient on if and how the patient would like the family to be involved. Despite being a new and junior member of staff, it is important to get your voice heard at the case conference and to share your observations with your team, as failing to do so will compromise the patient's well-being.

The nurse and the team as a whole in this scenario could consider other novel ways of sharing information between other professional groups, other than the case conference, using information and communication technology, for example. It is increasingly popular to use social media as a means of sharing information between professionals to promote shared interprofessional decision making and sharing responsibilities for care across team members (McNab, 2009). For example, doctors in a Canadian hospital were assigned individual and team smartphones with which they could contact each other and share information. Nurses and other staff could make direct calls or send e-mail messages to team smartphones via an online webpage site from computers on the wards. Although not without complications, this was successful in helping transmit information between doctors, nurses and other medical staff (Lo et al., 2012).

Patient-centred care

Health and social care practitioners should be able to seek out, integrate and value, as a partner, the input and the engagement of the patient and family (Orchard and Bainbridge, 2010).

This competency highlights why the narrower definition of interprofessional working has been expanded from *how two or more professionals may work together effectively in the interests of continuous care and the patient* (Freeth et al., 2002) to one that includes the older person and family. The patient and family should be seen as part of the team, centrally involved in common goal setting and shared decision making. In other words, interprofessional working should be defined as a range of different professionals *working with patients, their families, carers and communities to deliver the highest quality of care across settings* (World Health Organization, 2010a, p. 13). This is in keeping with a humanistic approach to care that puts an emphasis on the lived experience and personal history of the older patient, embodying the life goals and values of the patient, rather than a professional-focused definition of problem-based care. The older person should be considered as part of the interprofessional team rather than its object. If interprofessional teams are to include the patient's voice then practitioners must try to understand the values, priorities and perspectives of the older person (Clark, 1995).

Activity 10.3 *Critical thinking*

Read case study part 1 again. Why is it that Charlotte does not appear to cooperate with the services offered to her?

An outline answer is provided at the end of the chapter.

Health and social care professionals should view Charlotte and her family as an integral part of the interprofessional team and include them in the planning and implementation of services or care. Mary has shown that she understands the complexity of her mother's needs beyond just her physical well-being. When Charlotte was still at home, Mary contacted a number of charities and public-sector organisations to help Charlotte with her garden; she had explored a befriending service to counteract Charlotte's loneliness and had researched the benefits available to support these services. Mary was able to give those supporting Charlotte greater insight into her needs and acted as a key gatekeeper, coordinating the numerous agencies which visited her mother.

Nurses and all health and social care professionals should share information with patients and their carers in a respectful manner. They should do so in a way that is understandable, allows discussion and promotes shared decision making. The GP, for example, in the consultation after Charlotte's fall, should share information with Mary and Charlotte in a way that allows them both to engage as equals in the consultation.

As a nurse you will consider the education the patient and their family may require. As Charlotte has not been responsible for the finances in her married life, she will need additional support to help her understand the allowances and benefits available to her, how to claim them and what services these may purchase. This is particularly relevant in the UK with the increased personalisation of health and social care services, and the award of individual budgets managed by the client/patient (Department of Health, 2005; Forder et al., 2012).

Health and social care professionals should listen respectfully to the expressed needs of all parties in shaping and delivering care or services. Mary and Charlotte both have needs to be considered. Mary's relationship with Charlotte is a complex one. Mary has many competing commitments, with a husband and disabled son who also require her attention. Before Charlotte entered hospital, Mary found caring for her mother tiring and frustrating. Her physical and emotional well-being should be taken into account when engaging her in Charlotte's care. If this is not compromised, she is a valuable member of the team.

Interprofessional role clarification

Healthcare professionals should understand their own role and the roles of those in other professions, and use this knowledge appropriately to establish and achieve better patient outcomes (Orchard and Bainbridge, 2010).

Case study part 4: the hospital experience

Mary visited Charlotte regularly when she was in hospital. She reported the wards as being understaffed, although the nursing staff did what they could to make Charlotte comfortable. Most of the patients on Charlotte's unit were elderly and in need of a high degree of care. On a number of occasions, when visiting, the wards smelled of urine and worse. Some patients wandered around wearing only gowns which were ill-fitting and undignified. There were individual mobile side trays at every bed with food and drinks which remained there for a considerable time. Charlotte had a yoghurt drink and a ham sandwich on her tray at one afternoon visiting session, which was still untouched during the evening visit. No attempt seemed to have been made to assist her to drink or eat, nor to give her water to keep her hydrated. She incurred a urinary tract infection as a result and became delirious and somewhat unmanageable.

Activity 10.4 — *Critical thinking*

Whose role was it to help Charlotte with her eating and drinking? Who was monitoring her nutrition and hydration?

An outline answer is provided at the end of the chapter.

In case study part 4, we reject the negative assumption that none of the health professionals on the ward had cared sufficiently to check that Charlotte had been fed. It is far more likely that, under the pressure of a very busy ward, everyone assumed that it was someone else's role and responsibility, leaving Charlotte neglected as a result. Understanding one's own and other professionals' roles and responsibilities is not always as easy as it might seem. With increased interprofessional working, boundaries between professional roles and responsibilities can become blurred, leading to confusion about who should perform a particular task and when. The blurring of boundaries between the role of the healthcare assistant (HCA) and nurse is a typical example of this. HCAs and other assistant practitioners (APs) were introduced to fill the gaps in the nursing NHS workforce, and free up nursing time for more specialised tasks. The introduction of these roles is what Nancarrow and Borthwick (2005) call vertical role substitution, in which tasks traditionally done by nurses were delegated to a less-qualified professional, the HCA. Horizontal substitution can also occur when roles are interchangeable between professionals of similar training level.

Vertical substitution is illustrated in a study by Thornley (2000) who, in exploring the perceived roles of the HCA, showed a large overlap between the tasks these professionals were performing and those performed by registered nursing staff (see Table 10.1 for a list of tasks completed by HCAs that might be perceived as nursing tasks and the percentage of HCAs that are completing these tasks). Similarly, Wakefield et al. (2010), in a review of AP job descriptions, found that the boundaries between nurses' and APs' roles, such as the HCA, are blurred and claim that this lack of clarity over what the AP role is can cause conflict and confusion in practice.

Task	Percentage of HCAs performing this task
Talk to/reassure patients and relatives	97
Make beds	86
Help bathe patients	83
Telephone liaison	83
Monitor/record patient observations	82
Help feed patients	79
Obtain specimens	78
Help with catheter care	61
Participate in meetings about patient care	57
Dressing and wound care	57
Assist in drawing up care plans	43
Handle syringes/equipment	43
Help with drug administration	42
Clinical stock control	37
Invasive procedures	18
Take blood samples	11

Table 10.1: Nursing tasks completed by healthcare assistants (HCAs)

(Source: Thornley, 2000, p. 454)

In our case study, interprofessional communication between the HCA and nurse is essential in order for them to clarify their roles, in this case who should check that the patient is eating and whether she needs help to do so. The nurse and HCA need to reflect on their own and others' professional role and clarify who is accountable for each particular task. All professionals have competencies specific to their particular training but there are shared competencies also. Where competencies are unique to one profession, the other professions need the skills to be able to access these unique competencies through consultation or referral to these groups. This requires a level of humbleness and appreciation of the skills of other groups or alternatively the confidence and sometimes courage to seek advice. Perceived professional hierarchies within healthcare may also make this difficult. Serious errors in care occur, however, when a professional has lacked the confidence to speak up in emergency situations (Reid, 2012). Nurses also need to understand what competencies are shared, where there is potential overlap, potential for either horizontal or vertical substitution, and how these might be managed.

To avoid oversights, as described in this case scenario, nurses should be able to describe their own role and that of other professionals on the ward clearly and accurately. In this case scenario, the nurse should have been clear about who was responsible for ensuring that Charlotte ate her meal and kept hydrated. If an HCA is available to the team, the nurse might delegate this role to the HCA but would need to do so in such a way that the HCA agreed and was clear that this was a responsibility she/he was being expected to complete. Alternatively, if the HCA is otherwise engaged, the nurse may choose to 'muck in' and help with this task, whilst ensuring the nurse is communicating with the HCA that she/he is taking on this role with the HCA's permission and knowledge, so as not to offend or encroach on the HCA's role if not required.

Interprofessional conflict resolution

Health and social care professionals should be able to engage themselves and others actively, including the patient and family, in positively and constructively addressing disagreements as they arise (Orchard and Bainbridge, 2010).

Various reasons exist for conflict between professional groups (Orchard and Bainbridge, 2010). One relates to professionals not understanding each other's roles and accountability. Conflict may have arisen between the HCA and the nurse as to who was responsible for helping Charlotte eat her lunch, for example. Imagine how much worse it would be if Charlotte had died of starvation, as elderly hospital patients have done. The other reason relates to different members having different goals related to their different approaches to care as well as their own individual beliefs and philosophies. These different ways of viewing the world are what Clark (1995) refers to as different mind maps of the world. This is because different professional groups throughout their training are socialised in different ways, learning different rules and ways of practising that are peculiar to their professional training. The most obvious example is medicine and social work. In medical education there is an emphasis on the scientific basis of medicine and the biology of illness. Social work education, on the other hand, takes a more holistic approach to the client/patient, a less reductionist and more humanistic approach. These very different ways of approaching 'work' may lead to poor communication. We cannot resolve these differences through a change in philosophy. What we have to do is understand that other professionals have different perspectives on client care and that the contribution of each of these perspectives should be equally valued (Drinka and Clark, 2000).

Case study part 5

After a month in the hospital, the bed was needed and so the NHS arranged for Charlotte to move to a nursing home. Within ten days, Charlotte improved beyond recognition. She was eating and drinking well, regained mobility and was being cared for by staff who treated her with respect and dignity. Although her dearest wish was to return to her own flat, she was lucid enough to realise that this was not possible, that she needed a high degree of care and pain management and she seemed happy with her treatment at the nursing home. She was encouraged to join in with the variety of entertainment on offer at the home and on several occasions Mary arrived to find her laughing or singing with the other residents.

Charlotte passed away peacefully in the nursing home after two months. Mary knew that she and her family had done their best for her towards the end of her life and was grateful for the nursing home staff

(continued)

continued ...

for their care, support and kindness to her mother. They had kept the family informed every step of the way as to who had visited, changes in medication, what she was eating, whether she had managed to get up that day, when they were arranging a bath, massage, visit to the hairdresser, manicure, pedicure, and so on. Mary reported total communication and consultation on all levels from all the staff. 'It is so important to keep the family informed and involved with the care of their loved ones', says Mary.

Conflict arises not only between professional groups but also between the family, the patient and the healthcare team. Let us consider what each team member wanted as an outcome.

Charlotte wanted to be discharged from the hospital and return home. Charlotte's goal was to return to a familiar place in which she was comfortable. Her family and the medical team wanted her admitted into a care home. For Mary and the medical team the goal was to have Charlotte in a location where she could be cared for appropriately and be safe. In resolving professional–professional or professional–patient conflicts, you should acknowledge that conflict is not necessarily a bad thing. With different groups holding such different ways of looking at things and with the multitude of different skills and life experiences each individual has to offer, it is natural that different approaches to care exist. In fact, these different opinions add to the innovativeness and creativity of a team. However, professionals should anticipate situations where conflict may arise and develop strategies to deal with these. In the HCA–nurse conflict, for example, role ambiguity caused the conflict. This could be overcome through open transparent discussion between HCA and nursing staff about what tasks needed to be achieved and who was responsible for these. Good leadership is required to make it comfortable for both parties to work together to develop procedures which identify the causes of conflict early on and for processes to be put in place to resolve them. As transparency is essential in interprofessional communication, conflict resolution should take place in a neutral environment, free of blame, in which all are free to express their view and feel themselves to have had a voice, regardless of whether the resolution is in their favour or not. We have seen that conflict resolution usually involves good leadership, and it is to that competence that we now turn.

Interprofessional collaborative leadership

Healthcare professionals should understand and apply leadership principles that support collaborative practice. They should also be aware of the principles of shared decision making. They should be able to work collaboratively to determine who will provide group leadership in any given situation (Orchard and Bainbridge, 2010).

There are many models of leadership and different people and professional groups may view leadership very differently. Miller et al. (2001) identified, through observations of interprofessional teams in healthcare, three different *team philosophies of working* within them: a directive, integrative or elective philosophy.

A directive philosophy was frequently held by members of the medical profession and non-specialist nurses. It was characterised by a need for a hierarchy within a team and a clear leader. In contrast, an integrative philosophy described the views of team members who saw collaborative working and being a team player as central to interprofessional team working. Members understood the importance and complexity of communication and the need for effective discussion. This was a philosophy often held by therapy and social work professions. Lastly, the authors described an elective working philosophy demonstrated by professionals who prefer to work autonomously and refer to other professionals only when they perceive the need. Miller et al. (2001) used mismatches in these philosophies among members of the interprofessional team to explain team conflict and poor team outcomes. Imagine therefore the conflict that might arise in a team that contains a consultant from an accident and emergency department and a social worker, each with very different perspectives on team leadership. The former may be accustomed to crisis scenarios in which a clear leader is required, a leader who details and direct the tasks of the team as a whole. The social worker on the other hand may be accustomed to developing team tasks through joint decision making and consensus with all team members and the patient. Not vocalising these different expectations of leadership and team working and agreeing a way forward that is appropriate to the clinical case scenario bodes badly for effective interprofessional working.

To achieve some consensus on leadership in healthcare, the Clinical Leadership Competency Framework in the UK (Leadership Academy, 2011) was developed. This supports a model of shared or distributed leadership: *a universal model such that all clinicians can contribute to the leadership task where and when their expertise and qualities are relevant* (Leadership Academy, 2011, p. 6). The framework lists these leadership competencies as being able to demonstrate:

- the development of particular personal qualities (including self-awareness and continuous personal development);
- the ability to work with others (including building interprofessional relationships and encouraging the contribution of team members from other professional groups);
- the ability to manage services (including skills in planning and managing resources, people and performance);
- the ability to improve services (including being able to encourage improvement, innovation and organisational change);
- the ability to set future direction (including being able to apply professional knowledge and research evidence to support change and then evaluating its impact).

Activity 10.5 — *Critical thinking*

Write a case study of Charlotte's experience of the hospital ward, but where Charlotte's nurse demonstrates shared or distributed leadership.

An outline answer is provided at the end of the chapter.

The clinical leadership framework resonates with both 'altruistic' and 'servant leadership' models. In the former, the leadership competencies listed above are demonstrated in such a way that leaders of interprofessional teams are able to see beyond their own interests and that of their own professional group or organisation and *be willing to give up parts of their territories if necessary* in the interests of better interprofessional or interagency collaboration (Axelsson and Axelsson, 2009). In case study part 1, this would have been essential when the duties of age-related charities and public-sector services overlapped in the delivery of Charlotte's care.

Similarly, in 'servant leadership' models, leadership has *less to do with directing other people and more to do with serving their needs and in fostering the use of shared power in an effort to enhance effectiveness in the professional role* (Neill et al., 2007, p. 427). The nurse concerned would be demonstrating this servant leadership if she suggested an interactive debriefing session with HCA staff where they could reflect on the pressures faced by the HCA staff and explore all staff roles and responsibilities related to the nutrition and hydration of the patient.

Closely related to these models of leadership is the concept of 'interprofessional shared decision making', described as the *reciprocal flow of medical and personal information, [between individuals], discussion of preferences, wishes and options, conjoint deliberation and decision-making process* (Körner et al., 2012, p. 1). These processes should occur, first, between all the professionals involved in a patient's care, jointly agreeing together as a team a care plan for the patient. Second, these processes should also occur between each of these professionals and the patient (Körner et al., 2012). The decision to move Charlotte to a care home, for example, should be a three-way affair in which the 'preferences, wishes and options' of the hospital staff, the care home staff, Charlotte and her family are consulted and her move to the care home agreed collaboratively.

Interprofessional team functioning

Healthcare professionals should understand the principles of teamwork dynamics and group/team processes to enable effective interprofessional collaboration (Orchard and Bainbridge, 2010).

Nurses need insight into how teams form and function. Team working is a skill that has to be learned and practised; it does not come naturally to everyone. The most common model of team working is the *stages of group development* (Tuckman, 1965) and the concept of team roles (Belbin, 2012). In the team development model, team functioning and the behaviour of team members are described in terms of a team life cycle – forming, storming, norming, performing and adjourning.

In the forming phase, the team has newly come together, and members are getting to know each other. Skills related to interprofessional role clarification will be important here. In the storming phase, differing individual or professional views are shared, which will often lead to conflict. If the team is able to move past this phase, and not all teams are able to do so, the team enters a norming phase, where conflicts are resolved and new common ways of working as a team are agreed. The skills of conflict resolution, interprofessional communication, interprofessional leadership and shared decision making will be important in moving the team through into this phase of its life cycle. Once the interprofessional team has agreed its norms/rules, it enters the performing phase where members collaborate optimally under these agreed conditions.

This model helps the health or social care professional understand that teams are units that need to be actively developed as they pass from one phase to the next. However, the model rests on the premise that teams arc fairly stable and identifiable structures. The professsionals from the range of services supporting Charlotte, when she was living at home, might not describe themselves as a team but still need to collaborate. In the complex interagency, interprofessional organisation of health and social care services, the idea of a team and its functioning may be more fluid (Bleakley, 2012), with professionals coming together only temporarily around a particular task before disbanding again. Other models to understand team functioning in these instances are described elsewhere (Bleakley, 2012).

Another commonly used model to describe team functioning is that of Belbin's team roles that propose that individuals within a team have a tendency towards playing one (or sometimes several) of nine main roles, each of which contributes to the success of the team (**www.belbin.com**). A team will work best if a balance of roles is achieved within it. When working as an interprofessional team member, therefore, health or social care professionals should regularly reflect on the functioning of this team, considering the phase of its development and the differing roles that different members are fulfilling, whether a balance has been achieved and if not, whether roles need to be altered or new staff introduced to take these functions. For example, one of the nine team roles is that of coordinator, described by Belbin as a mature, confident individual, who is a good chairperson, who clarifies goals, promotes decision making and delegates well. This role is particularly important in the coordination of an interprofessional team. Although this role may be filled by one of the healthcare professionals, Begun et al. (2011) suggest that interprofessional teams import healthcare administrators to perform this function, leaving other roles to be fulfilled by other team members.

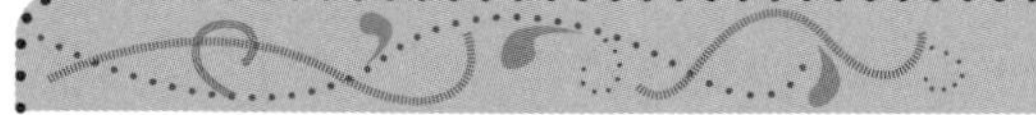

Chapter summary

This chapter explored the increasing need for interprofessional working in the healthcare of an ageing population. It presented the most up-to-date and international definition of interprofessional collaboration and outlined six competencies that healthcare professionals must develop if they are to deliver best interprofessional care for an older patient. The first of these competencies is the ability to communicate across professional and organisational boundaries and with different patient groups. This involves an awareness that other groups communicate in different ways and that one's own communication strategies need to adapt to take this into account.

The patient and family must be at the centre of the interprofessional team and be engaged as active team members in shared decision making. Active listening is key. Health and social care professionals need to be able to describe their own role and that of others. They should recognise the unique competencies of others, as well as where role overlap may cause confusion about who does what and when. Conflict resolution is a normal and central skill in working interprofessionally around an older patient and some of the reasons for interprofessional conflict are highlighted. Shared or distributed interprofessional leadership is important in the functioning of an interprofessional team, and models that promote servant or altruistic leadership styles and interprofessional shared decision making are preferred. Finally, two common models of team functioning are highlighted that enable the professional to reflect and act on how team processes may be explained and improved.

Activities: brief outline answers

Activity 10.1

Mary enlisted a large number of organisations to help her mother. GPs, district nurses and social workers from the public sector will all need to interact and collaborate with qualified professionals (potentially social workers and healthcare professionals) as well as volunteers in the third sector (e.g. Age UK) or religious leaders (from local religious groups). Collaboration, with Charlotte at its centre, is therefore required between a range of very distinct groups who vary by sector, professional group and professional status.

Mary plays a key coordination role in her mother's care. She has a holistic view of Charlotte's needs that is not confined to her poor physical health alone. Through her experience with her son, she has a good knowledge of the range of services and support available and how to access these and she is able to draw together a wide range of services, from gardening and cleaning services to health and social care. Mary and Charlotte are vital members of this broad team of people supporting them, as they hold vital information on who is doing what and how. Professionals should use this information to prevent duplication or oversights in the multiple services provided and to enable the different organisations and professionals to collaborate better in the interest of the patient.

Activity 10.2

Poor communication has occurred between different organisations when Mary is referred between one service and another and a mix-up in appointments has occurred. More seriously, there has been confusion around what can be done about Charlotte's prolapse. Mary's story suggests that different professionals have not shared or agreed a common approach to her condition, leading to Charlotte being confused and distressed. Poor communication is reported also in the GP consultation when Charlotte had cut her back. If Mary had not been there as an advocate, Charlotte may have left, not wanting to be a nuisance or make a fuss, and have withheld that she would not be able to apply the cream by herself.

Activity 10.3

Charlotte comes from a generation where privacy was highly valued. She may find asking for help from strangers uncomfortable. A befriending service may be a good idea to both Mary and the other professionals but for Charlotte it may be seen as undignified and intrusive. Professionals should consider these intergenerational differences and consult the patient on his or her personal preferences. In other words, they should try to understand the mind map of their older patient.

Activity 10.4

NHS careers (**http://www.nhscareers.nhs.uk/explore-by-career/wider-healthcare-team/careers-in-the-wider-healthcare-team/clinical-support-staff/healthcare-assistant**) describe the role of the HCA, as defined by washing and dressing, feeding, helping people to mobilise, toileting, bed making, generally assisting with patients' overall comfort and monitoring patients' condition by taking temperatures, pulse, respirations and weight. This suggests that it may have been the responsibility of the HCA to help Charlotte eat and hydrate, but research by Wakefield et al. (2010) and Thorley (2000) indicates that differentiating roles between the groups can be difficult and this may have led to Charlotte being neglected in this way.

Activity 10.5

The nurse on Charlotte's ward could demonstrate interprofessional leadership by proactively engaging medical, fellow nursing staff, and APs in a service improvement project aimed at improving the dignity of older people on her ward. After actively listening to Mary's account of experiences of the ward cleanliness, she decides to focus on the personal hygiene domain of the dignity framework, described in a recent report she is reading (Magee et al., 2008). She reads regularly as part of her own professional development as a nurse. She works collaboratively to plan, implement and evaluate a strategy in which staff offer patients choice in the level of assistance in personal hygiene they require, as well as who delivers it. They offer patients the choice of using their own toiletries and take extra measures to ensure the bathroom facilities on the ward are clean and welcoming. The nurse evaluates the impact of the project on patient experiences of the ward.

Useful websites

Centre for the Advancement of Interprofessional Education: www.caipe.org.uk

IPE PORTAL on MedEd for interprofessional education and practice articles and research: https://www.mededportal.org/ipe

Theoretical frameworks in interprofessional education and practice: http://www.facebook.com/groups/IN2THEORY

Further reading

Hammick, M, Freeth, DS, Goodsman, D and Copperman, J (2009) *Being Interprofessional.* Cambridge: Polity Press.

Glossary

Adaptive/maladaptive strategies Strategies or ways in which people do things that are either helpful and do not cause them extra problems (adaptive) or that do cause them extra problems (maladaptive).

Agency A person's ability to act or do something.

Autonomy A simple description reflecting the ability of an individual to make an informed choice without any form of coercion, usually with regard to choices to be made regarding the person's life and current circumstances.

Black and minority ethnic (BME) groups Minority ethnic groups are all groups excluding white British.

Culture Symbolic concept that embodies values, lifestyles, manners, customs, food and dress and is connected with the construction of group boundaries.

Dehumanisation Process by which people are removed of their personhood and simply seen as objects or tasks.

Directive Philosophies of leadership and team working characterised by a need for a hierarchy within a team and a clear leader.

Discrimination Treating a person or group differently (often negatively) because of a particular attribute such as age, race or sexuality.

Disempowerment A process by which people are deprived of power and choices regarding their lives and treatment.

Elective Philosophies of leadership and team working characterised by professionals who prefer to work autonomously and who refer to other professionals only when they perceive the need.

Emic Internal perspective of something or someone.

Emotion-focused Where feelings are focused on or are the central point.

Emotional isolation Commonly described as when individuals feel there is a lack of intimacy and meaningful attachments within their life.

Equality When everyone has the same or nearly similar chances to achieve their goals.

Essentialism The belief that social differences are determined by biology.

Ethnicity Actual or perceived common ancestry, language and regional or national origin.

Ethnocentrism Judging other cultures by the standards of our own on the understanding that our own culture is superior.

Etic External judgement of something or someone.

Homogeneous Simply put, this means alike or of the same kind. The assumption is that everyone within a particular social group are all the same and have the same interests.

Horizontal substitution This occurs when roles are interchangeable between professionals of similar training level.

Humanisation A framework designed to help ensure that all those we care for are treated as human beings.

Humanising values framework A structure for care that focuses on what is important to the individual as a human being.

Infantilisation A process in which adults are treated as if they are children.

Integrative Philosophies of leadership and team working characterised by views that collaborative working and being a team player are central to interprofessional team working.

Loneliness An awareness and discomfort due to a lack of social support or contact.

Mind maps Diagrams exploring different ways of viewing the world.

Monotonous Always the same, not exciting, boring.

Organic Of or relating to living matter. In this context, ill health that has a physiologically identifiable cause.

Paternalistic Thinking that you know what is best for individuals and therefore not consulting with them or enabling them to have a choice regarding their life; making decisions for others without consulting them.

Private sector Organisations funded privately (e.g. private healthcare companies).

Problem-focused Dealing with a challenge or difficulty by attempting to resolve it.

Psychometric tests Assessments or measurements of psychological functioning which can involve personality, intelligence or illness.

Public sector Organisations funded by the state (e.g. social services).

'Race' The scientific concept, not now accepted, of the ability to divide up humans on the basis of their different physical attributes.

Racism Attitude that one 'race' (group perceived as different based on appearance or place of origin) is superior or inferior to another.

Recovery approach The focus of care or support on the process individuals go through/the journey they take to move forward with their life to return to a state of well-being.

Shared or distributed leadership A model in which all can contribute to the leadership task where and when their expertise and qualities are relevant.

Social exclusion Where a person or group of people cannot access the opportunities or rights that are generally available to the society they live in, including housing, education and employment.

Social inclusion The positive effects of those measures that are taken to result in a change in circumstances and/or habits that mitigate against social exclusion, thus enabling people or communities to participate fully and meaningfully in society (**http://www.charitycommission.gov.uk/media/95497/socinc.pdf**).

Social isolation Commonly described as an objective assessment of an individual's social network, where there are perceived to be few actual contacts or opportunities to meet others and little involvement in community life or the wider social environment. It can also be used to infer living arrangements (e.g. living alone) or the lack of friends.

Solitude A term commonly used to describe the positive state of being alone by choice, for the purposes of inner reflection and enjoyment.

Stereotyping Assuming that individuals are the same as others in their social group, e.g. all older people are the same because they are old, and therefore have the same attributes (e.g. confusion, incontinence) or enjoy the same activities (e.g. bingo).

Subjective A view or way of looking at something based on an individual's personal feelings, tastes or opinions.

Third sector Not-for-profit organisations, often with charitable body status; also called the voluntary sector, e.g. age-related charities.

Vertical role substitution Occurs when tasks traditionally done by one profession are delegated to less qualified professionals.

Visuospatial The visual processing of the relationship between objects, the space between them. How people see objects within the environment.

Welfarism Process by which individuals are automatically assumed to require assistance simply because they are old or have a disability.

References

Abley, C, Bond, J and Robinson, L (2011) Improving interprofessional practice for vulnerable older people: Gaining a better understanding of vulnerability. *Journal of Interprofessional Care* 1–7.

Achenbaum, W (2005) Chapter 1: Ageing and changing: International historical perspectives on ageing. In: Johnson, M (ed.) *The Cambridge Handbook of Age and Ageing*. Cambridge: Cambridge University Press.

Action on Elder Abuse (2003) *Defining Abuse*. Available from: http://www.elderabuse.org.uk/Mainpages/Abuse/abuse.html (accessed 12 November 2012).

Adamson, K (2011) *Interprofessional Empathy in an Acute Healthcare Setting*. Theses and Dissertations (Comprehensive), paper 1119. Available from: http://scholars.wlu.ca/etd/1119 (accessed 1 December 2012).

Age Concern (2001) *'Opening Doors': Older lesbian and gay people – forgotten no more*. London: Age Concern.

Age Concern (2006) *Hungry to be Heard*. London: Age Concern.

Age Concern (2008) *Out of Sight, Out of Mind: Social exclusion behind closed doors*. London: Age Concern. Available from: http://image.guardian.co.uk/sys-files/Society/documents/2008/02/15/outofsight.pdf (accessed 2 September 2013).

Age Concern (2010) *Later Matters: Tacking race inequalities in BME older people*. Sheffield: Age Concern.

Age Concern (2011) *Forced Retirement*. Available from http://www.ageuk.org.uk/work-and-learning/discrimination-and-rights/default-retirement-age---frequently-asked-questions/ (accessed August 2013).

Age Concern (2012) *Falls Prevention*. Available from: http://www.ageuk.org.uk/health-wellbeing/keeping-fit/preventing-falls (accessed 2 September 2013).

Age UK (2010a) *Loneliness and Isolation Evidence Review*. London: Age UK.

Age UK (2010b) *Still Hungry to be Heard*. London: Age UK.

Age UK (2012) *Stop Falling: Start saving lives and money*. London: Age UK.

Ahmad, W and Bradby, H (2008) Ethnicity and health: Key themes in a developing field. *Current Sociology*, 56 (1): 47–56.

Alabaster, E (2007) Involving students in the challenges of caring for older people. *Nursing Older People*, 19 (6): 23–28.

Almeida, OP and Almeida, SA (1999). Short versions of the Geriatric Depression Scale: A study of their validity for the diagnosis of a major depressive episode according to the ICD-10 and DSM-IV. *International Journal of Geriatric Psychiatry*, 14: 858–865.

Alzheimer's Society (2009) *Counting the Cost: Caring for people with dementia on hospital wards.* Available from: http://alzheimers.org.uk/site/scripts/download_info.php?fileID=787 (accessed 2 September 2013).

Alzheimer's Society (2012) Demography. Available from: http://alzheimers.org.uk/site/scripts/documents_info.php?documentID=412 (accessed 2 September 2013).

American Psychiatric Association (2011) *DSM-IV-TR, The current manual.* Arlington, VA: American Psychiatric Association.

Anderson, G (2010) Loneliness amongst older adults aged 45+. AARP Magazine. Knowledge Networks and Insight Policy Research. Available from: http://assets.aarp.org/rgcenter/general/loneliness_2010.pdf (accessed 2 September 2013).

Andrade, M and Knight, J (2008) Exploring the anatomy and physiology of ageing. Part 4. The renal system. *Nursing Times,* 104 (34). Available from: www.nursingtimes.net (accessed 2 September 2013).

Axelsson, SB and Axelsson, R (2009) From territoriality to altruism in interprofessional collaboration and leadership. *Journal of Interprofessional Care,* 23 (4): 320–330. Available from: http://www.ncbi.nlm.nih.gov/pubmed/19517284 (accessed 5 December 2012).

Barker, P (2005) Editorial: Vulnerability. *Whitireia Nursing Journal,* 12: 5–8.

Barker, S (2007) *Vital Notes for Nurses: Psychology*. Oxford: Blackwell Publishing.

Barker, S (2011) *Midwives' Emotional Care of Women Becoming Mothers*. Newcastle upon Tyne: Cambridge Scholars.

Barker, S and Board, M (2012) *Dementia Care in Nursing.* London: Sage/Learning Matters.

Barker, W (2013) Practice question: Falls prevention services. *Nursing Older People,* 25 (5): 12.

Barry, A and Yuill, C (2008) *Understanding the Sociology of Health: An Introduction,* 2nd edn. London: Sage.

Barton, D and May, AL (2012) *Adult Nursing: Preparing for practice.* London: Hodder Arnold.

Bartram, D (2005) *Excluded Older People: New policy approaches.* Social Exclusion Unit. Presentation at the W and SW Regional Housing LIN, Weston-Super-Mare, 21 July 2005.

Batchelor, D (2006) Vulnerable voices: An examination of the concept of vulnerability in relation to student voice. *Educational Philosophy and Theory,* 38 (6): 787–800.

Beattie, A, Daker-White, G, Gillard, J and Means, R (2004) How can they tell? A qualitative study of the views of younger people about their dementia and dementia care services. *Health and Social Care in the Community,* 12: 359–368.

Begun, JW, White, KR and Mosser, G (2011) Interprofessional care teams: the role of the healthcare administrator. *Journal of Interprofessional Care,* 25 (2): 119–123. Available from: http://www.ncbi.nlm.nih.gov/pubmed/20846046 (accessed 6 December 2012).

Belbin, RM (2012) *Belbin Team Roles.* Available from: www.belbin.com (accessed 1 December 2012).

Benner, PE (1984) *From Novice to Expert: Excellence and power in clinical nursing practice.* Menlo Park, CA: Addison Wesley.

Best, C and Evans, L (2013) Identification and management of patients' nutritional needs. *Nursing Older People,* 25 (3): 30–36.

Betts Adams, K, Roberts, AR and Cole, MB (2011) Changes in activity and interest in the third and fourth age associations with health, functioning and depressive symptoms. *Occupational Therapy International,* 18 (1): 4–17.

Biley, F, Hilton, W, Phillips, J and Board, M (2011) A brief report on an action learning group exploration of how older people adapt to change in later life. *Nursing Reports,* 1: 1–20.

Birren, J (2007) *The Encyclopedia of Gerontology,* 2nd edn. Amsterdam: Academic Press.

Black's Medical Dictionary 42nd edn (2010) Available from: http://www.credoreference.com/entry/blackmed/ageing (accessed 8 April 2013).

Bleakley, A (2012) Working in 'teams' in an era of 'liquid' healthcare: What is the use of theory? *Journal of Interprofessional Care,* May: 1–9. Available from: http://www.ncbi.nlm.nih.gov/pubmed/22780569 (accessed 9 November 2012).

Boldy, N and Grenade, L (2008) Social isolation and loneliness among older people: Issues and future challenges in community and residential settings. *Australian Health Review,* 32 (3): 468–478.

Bornat, J and Bytheway, B (2010) Perceptions and presentations of living with everyday risk in later life. *British Journal of Social Work,* 40 (4): 1118–1134.

Bournemouth Echo (2010) Highlighting plight of isolated elderly people. Saturday 2 January.

Bowers, B (2009) Students must not underestimate the value of giving personal care. *Nursing Times,* 105 (43): 9.

Bowling, A and Gabriel, Z (2007) Lay theories of quality of life in older age. *Ageing and Society,* 27 (6): 827–848.

Branning, M (2011) Aging and *C. difficile* infection: The immune and gastrointestinal impact. *Gastrointestinal Nursing,* 9 (4): 42–47.

Bridges, J, Flatley, M, Meyer, J and Nicholson, C (2009) *Best Practice for Older People in Acute Care Settings: Guidance for nurses.* London: RCN.

Bridges, J, Flatley, M and Meyer, J (2010) Older people's and relatives' experiences in acute care settings: Systematic review and synthesis of qualitative studies. *International Journal of Nursing Studies,* 47 (1): 89–107.

British Heart Foundation Statistical Database (2010) *Ethnic Differences in Cardiovascular Disease.* Available at: http://www.bhf.org.uk/plugins/PublicationsSearchResults/DownloadFile.aspx?docid=a60f60ea-3c48-4632-868f-1fcfd00e088f&version=-1&title=Ethnic+Differences+in+Cardiovascular+Disease&resource=HS2010ED (accessed 2 September 2013).

Brocklehurst, H and Laurenson, M (2008) A concept analysis examining the vulnerability of older people. *British Journal of Nursing,* 17 (21): 1354–1357.

Brown, A and Draper, P (2003) Accommodative speech and terms of endearment: Elements of a language mode often experienced by older adults. *Journal of Advanced Nursing,* 41 (1): 15–21.

Brown, J, Nolan, M, Davies, S, Nolan, J and Keady, J (2008) Transforming students' views of gerontological nursing: Realising the potential of 'enriched' environments of learning and care: A multi-method longitudinal study. *International Journal of Nursing Studies,* 45 (8): 1214–1232.

Brownie, S and Horstmanshof, L (2011) The management of loneliness in aged care residents: An important therapeutic target for gerontological nursing. *Geriatric Nursing,* 32 (5): 318–325.

Brunner, E (1997) Socioeconomic determinants of health: Stress and the biology of inequality. *British Medical Journal,* 314: 7092.

Bytheway, B (1995) *Ageism.* Buckingham: Open University Press.

Cacioppo, JT (2002) Social neuroscience: Understanding the pieces fosters understanding the whole and vice versa. *American Psychologist,* 57: 819–830.

Canton, N, Clark, C and Pietka, E (2008) *'The Thing Is That We Haven't Come Here for Holidays': The experiences of new migrant communities from Central and Eastern Europe who are living and working in Glasgow.* Edinburgh: British Council and the Institute for Public Policy Research.

Care Quality Commission (2011) *Dignity and Nutrition, Inspection Programme: National overview.* Newcastle: Care Quality Commission.

Cartwright, C, Hughes, M and Lienert, T (2012) End-of-life care for gay, lesbian, bisexual and transgender people. *Culture, Health and Sexuality,* 14 (5): 537–548.

Cattan, M (2011) *Isolation Week.* Available from: http://www.emeraldinsight.com/journals.htm?articleid=17009829&show=html (accessed 2 September 2013).

Cattan, M, Newell, C, Bond, J and White, M (2003) Alleviating social isolation and loneliness among older people. *International Journal of Mental Health Promotion,* 5 (3): 20–30.

Cattan, M, Bond, J, Learmouth, A and White, M (2005) Preventing social isolation and loneliness among older people: A systematic review of health promotion interventions. *Ageing and Society,* 25 (1): 41–67.

Clare, L (2002) We'll fight it as long as we can: Coping with the onset of Alzheimer's disease. *Aging and Mental Health,* 6: 139–148.

Clark, PG (1995) Quality of life, values and teamwork in geriatric care: do we communicate what we mean? *Gerontologist,* 35: 402–411.

Cohen, S, Doyle, WJ, Skoner, DP, Rabin, BS and Gwaltney, JM, Jr (1997) Social ties and susceptibility to the common cold. *Journal of the American Medical Association,* 277: 1940–1944.

Collins, S (2009) Good communication helps to build a therapeutic relationship. *Nursing Times,* 105 (24): 11.

Commission on Dignity in Care for Older People (2012) *Delivering Dignity: Securing dignity in care for older people in hospitals and care homes.* London: Commission on Dignity in Care, a collaboration established by the NHS Confederation, the Local Government Association and Age UK. Available from http://tinyurl.com/cque4ox (accessed 12 November 2012).

Cornell Institute for Translational Research on Aging. *Social Isolation: Strategies for Connecting and Engaging Older People.* Available from: http://www.cornell.edu/search/index.cfm?tab=&q=citra (accessed 2 September 2013).

Cornman, JC, Goldman, N, Glei, DA, Weinstein, M and Chang, MC (2003) Social ties and perceived support: Two dimensions of social relationships and health among the elderly in Taiwan. *Journal of Aging and Health*, 15: 616–644.

Cornwell, EY and Waite, L (2009) Social disconnectedness, perceived isolation, and health among older adults. *Journal of Health and Social Behavior*, 50 (1): 31–48.

Cornwell, J (2012) *The Care of Frail Older People with Complex Needs: Time for a revolution.* The Sir Roger Bannister Health Summit, March 2012. Leeds Castle: The King's Fund.

Craig, C, Atkin, K, Chattoo, S and Flynn, R (2012) *Understanding 'Race' and Ethnicity.* Bristol: Policy Press.

Crawford, K and Walker, J (2003) *Social Work and Human Development*, 2nd edn. Exeter: Learning Matters.

Cronin, A and King, A (2010) Power, inequality and identification: Exploring diversity and intersectionality amongst older LGB adults. *Sociology*, 44: 876–891.

Cruickshank, M (2003) *Learning to Be Old: Gender, culture and aging.* Lanham, MD: Rowman and Littlefield.

Cummings, J (2012) Jane Cummings' voicepiece. *Chief Nursing Officer Bulletin*, May: 1–2.

Cummings, J (2013) *Nursing Vision.* Available from: http://www.england.nhs.uk/nursingvision/ (accessed 26 June 2013).

Cupples, ME (2012) Improving healthcare access for people with visual impairment and blindness. *British Medical Journal*, 344: e542.

De Jong-Gierveld, J (1987) Developing and testing a model of loneliness. *Journal of Personality and Social Psychology*, 53: 119–128.

Department of Health (2000) *No Secrets.* London: HMSO.

Department of Health (2001a) *Essence of Care.* Available from: http://www.dh.gov.uk/en/Publicationsandstatistics/Publications/PublicationsPolicyAndGuidance/DH_4005475 (accessed 2 September 2013).

Department of Health (2001b) *National Service Framework for Older People.* Available from: http://webarchive.nationalarchives.gov.uk/+/www.dh.gov.uk/en/Publicationsandstatistics/Publications/PublicationsPolicyAndGuidance/Browsable/DH_4901314 (accessed 8 April 2013).

Department of Health (2001c) *The Journey to Recovery: The government's vision for mental health care.* London: Department of Health. Available from: http://www.dh.gov.uk/prod_consum_dh/groups/dh_digitalassets/@dh/@en/documents/digitalasset/dh_4058900.pdf (accessed 2 September 2013).

Department of Health (2002) *Fair Access to Care Services: Guidance for eligibility criteria for adult social care.* London: Department of Health.

Department of Health (2005) *Independence, Well-Being and Choice.* London: Department of Health.

Department of Health (2006) *Our Health, Our Care, Our Say: New direction for community services: A brief guide.* London: Department of Health.

Department of Health (2007a) *Commissioning Framework for Health and Wellbeing.* Available from: http://www.dh.gov.uk/prod_consum_dh/groups/dh_digitalassets/documents/digitalasset/dh_072605.pdf (accessed 2 September 2013).

Department of Health (2007b) *National Service Framework for Older People.* London: DH. Available from: http://www.dh.gov.uk/en/Publicationsandstatistics/Publications/PublicationsPolicyAndGuidance/Browsable/DH_4096710 (accessed 2 September 2013).

Department of Health (2008) *No Patient Left Behind: How can we ensure world class primary care for black and minority ethnic people?* London: HMSO.

Department of Health (2009a) *Tackling Health Inequalities: 10 years on.* London: Department of Health.

Department of Health (2009b) *Living Well with Dementia: A national dementia strategy.* London: The Stationery Office.

Department of Health (2009c) *New Horizons. A shared vision for mental health.* London: Department of Health. Available from: http://www.dh.gov.uk/prod_consum_dh/groups/dh_digitalassets/@dh/@en/documents/digitalasset/dh_109708.pdf (accessed 2 September 2013).

Department of Health (2009d) *Safeguarding Adults: Report on the consultation on the review of 'No Secrets'.* London: HMSO.

Department of Health (2010a) *Inclusion Health: Improving primary care for socially excluded people.* London: The Stationery Office.

Department of Health (2010b) *Fair Society, Healthy Lives: The Marmot review: Executive summary.* London: Department of Health.

Department of Health (2010c) *Essence of Care.* London. Available from: https://www.gov.uk/government/uploads/system/uploads/attachment_data/file/216691/dh_119978.pdf (accessed 2 September 2013).

Department of Health (2011a) *Safeguarding Adults: The role of health service practitioners.* London: Department of Health.

Department of Health (2011b) *Common Principles for Supporting People with Dementia.* Available from: https://www.gov.uk/government/publications/common-core-principles-for-supporting-people-with-dementia (accessed 2 September 2013).

Department of Health (2012) *Public Health: Obesity.* Available from: http://www.dh.gov.uk/en/Publichealth/Obesity/index.htm (accessed 2 September 2013).

Department of Health and NHS Commissioning Board (2012) *Developing the Culture of Compassionate Care: Creating a new vision for nurses, midwives and care-givers.* London: Department of Health.

Department for Work and Pensions (2001) *The Pensioners' Income Series 1999/2000.* London: Department for Work and Pensions, Analytical Services Division.

Department for Work and Pensions (2008) *Working Together: UK national action plan on social inclusion 2008–2010.* London: Department of Work and Pensions.

D'Hondt, A, Kaasalainen, S, Prentice, D and Schindel Martin, L (2011) Bathing residents with dementia in long-term care: Critical incidents described by personal support workers. *International Journal of Older People Nursing,* 7 (4): 253–263.

Dickens, AP, Richards, S, Greaves, C and Campbell, J (2011) Interventions targeting social isolation in older people: A systematic review. *BMC Public Health,* 11: 647.

Diez Roux, AV (2001) Investigating neighbourhood and area effects on health. *American Journal of Public Health,* 91: 1783e9.

Doka, K (2002) *Disenfranchised Grief: New directions, challenges and strategies for practice.* Champaign, IL: Research Press.

Drennan, J, Treacy, MP, Butler, M, Byrne, A, Fealy, G and Frazer, K (2008) Support networks of older people living in the community. *International Journal of Older People Nursing,* 8: 234e42.

Drinka, T and Clark, PG (2000) *Health Care Team Work: Interdisciplinary practice and teaching.* Westport, CT: Auburn House.

Easterlin, RA (1987) New age structure of poverty in America: Permanent or transient? *Population and Development Review,* 13 (2): 195–208.

Easterlin, RA, Macdonald, C and Macunovich, DJ (1990) Retirement prospects of the baby boom generation. *Gerontologist,* 30 (6): 776–783.

Eastman, M (2008) Safeguarding vulnerable adults: Policy and practice update. In*: A Practical Guide to Safeguarding Vulnerable Adults. 5th International Conference.* London.

Egan, G (1975) *The Skilled Helper: A systematic approach to effective helping.* Pacific Grove, CA: Brooks/Cole.

Ellins, J (2012) *Understanding and Improving Transitions of Older People: A user and carer perspective.* London: National Institute for Health Research, NETSCC, HS&DR.

Emblin, K (2011) Community-based systems for medicines administration. *Nurse Prescribing,* 9 (7): 353–357.

European Economy (2012) *The 2012 Ageing Report: Economic and budgetary projections for the 27 Member States (2010–2060).* Joint report prepared by the European Commission (DG ECFIN) and the Economic Policy Committee (AWG). Available from: http://ec.europa.eu/economy_finance/publications/european_economy/2012/pdf/ee-2012-2_en.pdf (accessed 8 April 2013).

Fagerberg, I and Engstrom, G (2012) Care of the old: A matter of ethics, organization and relationships. *International Journal of Qualitative Studies on Health and Well-Being,* 7: 9684.

Faulkner, KA, Cauley, JA, Znuda, JM, Griffin, JM and Nevitt, MC (2003) Is social integration associated with the risk of falling in older community dwelling women? *Journals of Gernotology, Series A., Biological Sciences and Medical Sciences,* 58: M954–M959.

Fenton, S (1999) *Ethnicity: Racism, class and culture.* Basingstoke: Macmillan.

Fioto, B (2002) Social isolation: Important construct in community health. *Geriatric Nursing,* 23 (1): 53–55.

Flaskerud, J, and Winslow, B (1998) Conceptualizing vulnerable populations: Health-related research. *Nursing Research,* 47: 69–77.

Fletcher, J (2009) Identifying patients at risk of malnutrition: Nutrition screening and assessment. *Gastrointestinal Nursing,* 7 (5): 12–17.

Flynn, M (2012a) *South Gloucestershire Safeguarding Adults Board: Winterbourne View Hospital: A serious case review*. Available at: http://hosted.southglos.gov.uk/wv/report.pdf (accessed 14 August 2013).

Flynn, M (2012b) *Winterbourne View Hospital: A serious case review*. South Gloucestershire Council. Available from http://hosted.southglos.gov.uk/wv/report.pdf (accessed 13 November 2012).

Forder, J, Jones, K, Glendinning, C, Caiels, J, Welch, E, Baxter, K, Davidson, J et al. (2012) *Evaluation of the Personal Health Budget Pilot Programme*. London: Department of Health.

Francis, R (2009) *Independent Enquiry into Care Provided at the Mid Staffordshire Foundation NHS Trust*, vols. 1 and 2. London: The Stationery Office.

Francis, R (2011) *Independent Inquiry into Care Provided by Mid Staffordshire NHS Foundation Trust January 2005–March 2009*. London: Stationery Office.

Francis, R (2013) *Report of the Mid Staffordshire NHS Foundation Trust Public Enquiry*. London: The Stationery Office. Available from: http://www.midstaffspublicinquiry.com/report (accessed 2 September 2013).

Freeth, D, Hammick, M, Koppel, I, Reeves, S and Barr, H (2002) *A Critical Review of Evaluations of Interprofessional Education*. Occasional paper no. 2. London: LTSN-Centre for Health Sciences and Practices.

Galvin, K and Todres, L (2012) *Caring and Well-Being: A lifeworld approach*. Oxford: Routledge.

Gardner, I, Brooke, E, Ozanne, E and Kendig, H (1998) *Improving Social Networks: A research report*. Adelaide: Lincoln Gerontology Centre, La Trobe University.

Geriatric Medicine and Nursing Standard (2008) *Urinary Continence Management in Older People: Continence essential guide*. Middlesex: RCN Publishing.

Gillespie, LD, Robertson, MC, Gllespie, WJ, Sherrington, C, Gates, S, Clemson, LM and Lamb, SE (2012) *Interventions for Preventing Falls in Older People Living in the Community*. Cochrane Library 11: 1–420.

Glacken, M and Higgins, A (2008) The grief experiences of same-sex couples within an Irish context: Tacit acknowledgement. *International Journal of Palliative Nursing*, 14 (6): 297–302.

Glass, TA, Mendes de Leon, C, Marottolli, R and Berkman, L (1999) Population based study of social and productive activities as predictors of survival among elderly Americans. *British Medical Journal*, 319: 478–483.

Gleibs, IH, Haslam, C, Jones, JM, Haslam, A, McNeill, J and Connolly, H (2011) No country for old men? The role of a 'gentlemen's club' in promoting social engagement and psychological well-being in residential care. *Aging and Mental Health*, 15 (4): 456–466.

Goldstein, D (2012) Role of aging on innate responses to viral infections. *Journals of Gerontology. Series A: Biological Sciences and Medical Sciences*, 67 (3): 242–246.

Gopinath, B, Schneider, J, McMahon, CM, Burlutsky, G, Leeder, S and Mitchell, P (2013) Dual sensory impairment in older adults increases the risk of mortality: A population-based study. *PLOS ONE* 8 (3). Available from: www.plosone.org (accessed 2 September 2013).

Graham, H (2000) *Understanding Health Inequalities*. Buckingham: Oxford University Press.

Griffin, J (2010) *The Lonely Society*? London: Mental Health Foundation. Available from: http://its-services.org.uk/silo/files/the-lonely-society.pdf (accessed 2 September 2013).

Guardian (2011) Half of NHS hospitals failing to care for elderly. Available from: http://www.guardian.co.uk/society/2011/oct/13/nhs-hospitals-care-of-elderly (accessed 29 July 2013).

Hadjistavropoulos, T, Fitzgerald, T and Delbaere, K (2011) Reconceptualizing the role of fear of falling and balance confidence in fall risk. *Journal of Aging and Health,* 23 (1): 3–23.

Hajjar, ER, Cafiero, AC and Hanlon, JT (2007) Polypharmacy in elderly patients. *American Journal of Pharmacology,* 5 (4): 345–351.

Hall, B and Scragg, T (eds) (2012) *Social Work with Older People: Approaches to person-centred practice.* Maidenhead: McGraw Hill OUP.

Hall, S (2013) Chasing longevity. *National Geographic,* 233: 5.

Hammill, M (2009) *Social Isolation and Older Adults' Mental Health.* More than just practical needs: The befriending options for isolated, older people and the benefits of regular social interaction. Available from: www.contact-the-elderly.org.uk/.../Dr_Michelle_Hamills_handouts.pdf (accessed March 2010).

Haney, C (2003) Mental health issues in long-term solitary and 'supermax' confinement. *Crime and Delinquency,* 49: 124.

Harker, P and Hemingway, A (2003) Social issues which underlie childhood behaviour applicable to CHD risk in adulthood. In: *A Lifecourse Approach to CHD Prevention: Scientific and policy review.* London: The Stationery Office.

Havighurst, RJ (1961) Successful aging. *The Gerontologist,* 1: 8–13.

Hawkley, L and Caccioppo, C (2010) Loneliness matters: A theoretical and empirical review of consequences and mechanisms. *Annals of Behavioural Medicine,* 40 (2): 218–227.

Healthcare Commission (2009) *Investigation into Mid Staffordshire NHS Foundation Trust.* London: Healthcare Commission.

Heaslip, V and Board, M (2012) Does nurses' vulnerability affect their ability to care? *British Journal of Nursing,* 21 (15): 912–916.

Heath, H and Schofield, I (1999) *Healthy Ageing: Nursing older people.* London: Mosby.

Heenan, D (2010) Social capital and older people in farming communities. *Journal of Aging Studies,* 24: 40–46.

Help the Aged/RCN. (2008) *Dignity on the Ward: Working with older people from ethnic minorities.* London: Help the Aged.

Hemingway, A (2012) Can humanisation theory contribute to the philosophical debate in public health? *Public Health,* 126: 448–453.

Hemingway, A and Stevens, P (2011) Innovating to achieve sustainable wellbeing inside the built environment. *Perspectives in Public Health,* 131 (3): 117–118.

Hemingway, A, Scammell, J and Heaslip, V (2012) Humanising nursing care: A theoretical model. *Nursing Times,* 108 (40): 26–27.

Henry, M (2002) Descending into delirium. *American Journal of Nursing,* 102 (3): 49–56.

Hicks, T (2008) *Social Work Practice with Older Lesbians and Gay Men: Developing practice with older lesbians and gay men.* Exeter: Learning Matters.

Hill, K, Sutton, L and Cox, L (2009) *Managing Resources in Later Life: Older people's experience of change and continuity.* York: Joseph Rowntree Foundation.

Hoban, M, James, V, Pattrick, K, Beresford, P and Fleming, J (2011) *Voices on Well-Being: A report of research with older people.* Cardiff: WRVS.

Hole, K (2011) *Loneliness Compendium: Examples from research and practice.* JRF programme paper: Neighbourhood approaches to loneliness. Joseph Rowntree Foundation. Available from: http://www.jrf.org.uk/sites/files/jrf/loneliness-neighbourhoods-engagement-full.pdf (accessed 2 September 2013).

Holley, UA (2007) Social isolation: a practical guide for nurses assisting clients with chronic illness. *Rehabilitation Nursing,* 32 (2): 51–58.

Home Office (2010) *The Equality Act.* Available at: http://homeoffice.gov.uk/equalities/equality-act (accessed 2 September 2013).

Hopson, B and Adams, J (1976) Towards an understanding of transition. In: Adams, J, Hopson, B and Hayes, H (eds) *Transition: Understanding and managing personal change.* London: Martin Robertson and Co.

House, JS (2001) Social isolation kills, but how and why? *Psychosomatic Medicine,* 63: 273–274.

Independent (2011) A lethal lack of dignity for the elderly. Available from: http://www.independent.co.uk/voices/editorials/leading-article-a-lethal-lack-of-dignity-for-the-elderly-2288917.html (accessed 29 July 2013).

Institute of Alcohol Studies (2010) *Alcohol and the Elderly.* IAS factsheet. Available from: http://www.ias.org.uk/Alcohol-knowledge-centre/Alcohol-and-older-people.aspx (accessed 2 September 2013).

Jack, E (2011) *Social Isolation: A research study. Helping lonely people make friends.* Bournemouth University. Available from http://staffprofiles.bournemouth.ac.uk/display/publication46044 (accessed 2 September 2013).

Kaufman, G (2011) Polypharmacy in older adults. *Nursing Standard,* 25 (38): 49–55.

Keenan, B, Jenkins, C, Denner, L, Harries, M, Fawcett, K, Magill, L, Atkins, S and Miller, J (2011) Promoting mental health in older people admitted to hospitals. *Nursing Standard,* 25 (20): 46–56.

Kennedy, I (2001) *Learning from Bristol: The report of the public inquiry into children's heart surgery at the Bristol Royal Infirmary 1984–1995.* London: Department of Health.

Kiecolt-Glaser, JK, Garner, W, Speicher, C, Penn, GM, Holliday, J and Glaser, R (1984) Psychosocial modifiers of immunocompetence in medical students. *Psychosomatic Medicine,* 46 (1): 7–14.

Kings Fund (2008) *Seeing the Person in the Patient.* London: Kings Fund.

Kinney, A, Yeomans, LE, Martin Bloor, C and Sandler, RS (2005) Social ties and colorectal cancer screening among blacks and whites in North Carolina. *Cancer Epidemiology, Biomarkers and Prevention,* 14: 182–189.

Kitwood, T (1993) Person and process in dementia. *International Journal of Geriatric Psychiatry,* 8: 541–545.

Kitwood, T (1997) *Dementia Reconsidered: The person comes first.* Buckingham: Open University Press.

Knapp, M (2010) *Research Realities: How befriending services can aid older people's well-being.* Community care. Available from: http://www.communitycare.co.uk/Articles/08/07/2010/114872/how-befriending-services-can-aid-older-peoples-well-being.htm (accessed 2 September 2013).

Knight, J and Nigam, Y (2008a) Exploring the anatomy and physiology of ageing. Part 5. The nervous system. *Nursing Times,* 104 (35). Available from: www.nursingtimes.net (accessed 2 September 2013).

Knight, J and Nigam, Y (2008b) Exploring the anatomy and physiology of ageing. Part 10. Muscles and bone. *Nursing Times,* 104 (48). Available from: www.nursingtimes.net (accessed 2 September 2013).

Kobassa, S (1979) Stressful life events, personality and health: An inquiry into hardiness. *Journal of Personality and Social Psychology,* 37: 1–11.

Körner, M, Ehrhardt, H and Steger, A-K (2012) Designing an interprofessional training program for shared decision making. *Journal of Interprofessional Care,* July : 1–9. Available from: http://www.ncbi.nlm.nih.gov/pubmed/23151149 (accessed 19 November 2012).

Laming, WH (2003) *The Victoria Climbié Report.* London: The Stationery Office.

Laming, WH (2009) *The Protection of Children in England: A Progress Report.* London: The Stationery Office.

Larson, R (1978) Thirty years of research on the subjective well-being of older Americans. *Journal of Gerontology,* 33 (1): 109–125.

Leadership Academy (2011) *Clinical Leadership Competency Framework.* London: Department of Health.

Lee, M (2006) *Promoting Mental Health and Well-Being in Later Life.* A first report from the UK Inquiry into Mental Health and Well-Being in Later Life. London: Age Concern and Mental Health Foundation.

Lee, M (2007) *Improving Services and Support for Older People with Mental Health Problems.* The second report from the UK Inquiry into Mental Health and Well-Being in Later Life. London: Age Concern. Available from: http://www.nmhdu.org.uk/silo/files/inquiry-full-report.pdf (accessed 2 September 2013).

Liddle, J, Carlson, G and McKenna, K (2004) Using a matrix in life transition research. *Qualitative Health Research,* 14 (10): 1396–1417.

Liu, YE, While, AE, Norman, IJ and Ye, W (2012) Health professionals' attitudes toward older people and older patients: A systematic review. *Journal of Interprofessional Care,* 26 (5): 397–409. Available from: http://www.ncbi.nlm.nih.gov/pubmed/22780579 (accessed 21 November 2012).

Lo, V, While, AE, Norman, LJ and Ye, W (2012) The use of smartphones in general and internal medicine units: A boon or a bane to the promotion of interprofessional collaboration? *Journal of Interprofessional Care,* 26 (4): 276–282. Available from: http://www.ncbi.nlm.nih.gov/pubmed/22482742 (accessed 14 November 2012).

Lum, YS and Lightfoot, E (2003) The effect of health on retirement saving among older workers. *Social Work Research,* 27: 31–44.

Machielse, A (2006) Social isolation and the elderly: Causes and consequences. In: *2006 Shanghai International Symposium 'Caring for the Elderly',* workshop 'Community and care for the elderly'. Shanghai, 26–29 June 2006.

Macunovich, DJ, Easterlin, RA, Schaeffer, CM and Cummins, EM (1995) Echoes of the baby boom and bust: Recent and prospective changes in living alone among elderly widows in the United States. *Demography*, 32 (1): 17–28.

Magee, H, Parsons, S and Askham, J (2008) *Measuring Dignity in Care for Older People: A research report for Help the Aged.* Oxford: Picker Institute Europe.

Marmot, M (2010) *Fair Society, Healthy Lives: The Marmot review.* Available at: www.ucl.ac.uk/marmotreview (accessed 14 August 2013).

Martinsen, K (2006) *Care and Vulnerability.* Stockholm: Akribe.

McCrae, N, Murray, J, Banerjee, S, Huxley, P, Bhugra, D, Tylee, A and MacDonald, A (2005) They're all depressed aren't they? A qualitative study of social care workers and depression in older adults. *Aging and Mental Health*, 9: 508–516.

McCulloch, A (2009) Old age and mental health in the context of the lifespan: What are the key issues in the 21st century? In: Williamson, T (ed.) *The Older People's Mental Health Handbook.* Brighton: Pavilion Publishing.

McCusker, J, Cole, M, Abrahamowicz, M, Han, L, Podoba, JE and Ramman-Haddad, L (2001) Environmental risk factors for delirium in hospitalized older people. *Journal of the American Geriatrics Society*, 49 (10): 1327–1334.

McKeown, J, Clarke, A, Ingleton, C, Ryan, T and Repper, J (2010) The use of life story work with people with dementia to enhance person-centred care. *International Journal of Older People Nursing*, 5 (2): 148–158.

McLaren, L and Hawe, P (2005) Ecological perspectives in health research. *Journal of Epidemiology and Community Health*, 59: 6e14.

McNab, C (2009) What social media offers to health professionals and citizens. *Bulletin of the World Health Organization*, 87: 566. Available from: http://www.who.int/bulletin/volumes/87/8/09-066712/en/#.UMDDnCA4Dn4.mendeley (accessed 6 December 2012).

Mental Health Foundation (2012) *Mental Health A-Z Older People.* Available from: http://www.mental-health.org.uk/help-information/mental-health-a-z/O/older-people (accessed 2 September 2013).

Miles, R and Brown, M (2003) *Racism,* 2nd edn. London: Routledge.

Miller, C, Ross, N and Freeman, M (2001) *Inter Professional Education in Health Social Care.* London: Arnold Publications.

Mistry, R, Rosansky, J, McGuire, J, McDermott, C, Jarvik, L and UPBEAT Collaborative Group (2001) Social isolation predicts re-hospitalisation in a group of older American veterans enrolled via the UPBEAT programme: Unified psychogeriatric biopsychosocial evaluation and treatment. *International Journal of Geriatric Psychaitry*, 16: 950–959.

Moriarty, J, Meiling, K, Coomber, C, Rutter, D and Turner, M (2010) *Communication Training for Care Home Workers: Outcomes for older people, staff, families and friends.* London: Social Care Institute for Excellence.

Moriarty, J, Sharif, N and Robinson, J (2011) *SCIE Research Briefing 35: Black and minority ethnic people with dementia and their access to support and services.* Social Care Institute for Excellence. Available at: http://www.scie.org.uk/publications/briefings/briefing35 (accessed 2 September 2013).

Morris, G and Morris, J (2010) *The Dementia Care Workbook.* Berkshire: Open University Press.

Mountford, H (2010) Got a lot o' livin' to do: Opportunities for older workers in the global financial crisis. *Australian Bulletin of Labour,* 36 (3): 238–259.

Munnell, A, Muldoon, D and Sass, S (2009) *Recessions and Older Workers.* Issue brief 9-2. Chestnut Hill, MA: Centre for Retirement Research at Boston College.

Myall, B, Hine, D, Marks, A, Thorsteinnsson, E, Brechman-Toussaint, M and Samuels, C (2009) Assessing individual differences in perceived vulnerability in older adults. *Personality and Individual Differences,* 46: 8–13.

Nancarrow, S and Borthwick, AM (2005) Dynamic professional boundaries in the healthcare workforce. *Sociology of Health and Illness,* 27 (7): 897–919. Available from: http://www.ncbi.nlm.nih.gov/pubmed/16313522 (accessed 30 November 2012).

Narayanasamy, A, Clissett, P, Parumal, I, Thompson, D, Annasamy, A and Edge, R (2004) Responses to the spiritual needs of older people. *Journal of Advanced Nursing,* 48 (1): 6–16.

National Cancer Intelligence Network and Cancer Research UK (2009) *Cancer Incidence and Survival by Major Ethnic Group, England 2002–2006.* Available at: http://www.ncin.org.uk/home.aspx (accessed 2 September 2013).

National Health Service (2007) *Adult Psychiatric Morbidity in England, 2007.* The Information Centre for Health and Social Care. Available from: http://www.hscic.gov.uk/pubs/psychiatricmorbidity07 (accessed 2 September 2013).

National Institute for Health and Care Excellence (2006) *Nutrition Support in Adults.* Available from: http://www.nice.org.uk/CG32 (accessed 2 September 2013).

National Institute for Health and Clinical Excellence (2007) *Depression (Amended). Management of depression in primary and secondary care.* Available from: http://www.iappcare.com/uploadedfiles/NICEguidelineamended.pdf (accessed 2 September 2013).

National Institute for Health and Clinical Excellence (2008) *Mental Wellbeing and Older People, Physical Activity.* PH16. Available from: http://guidance.nice.org.uk/PH16 (accessed 2 September 2013).

National Institute for Health and Clinical Excellence (2011) *NHS: NICE and SCIE Guidelines for Dementia.* Available from: http://www.nice.org.uk/nicemedia/live/10998/30318/30318.pdf (accessed 2 September 2013).

National Institute for Health and Care Excellence (2013) *Falls: Assessment and prevention of falls in older people.* Available from: http://www.nice.org.uk/nicemedia/live/14181/64088/64088.pdf (accessed 2 September 2013).

Nay, R (2010) Guest editorial: Is care still the 'essence' of nursing? *International Journal of Older People,* 5 (3): 189–190.

Nazarko, L (2008) A guide to continence assessment for community nurses. *British Journal of Community Nursing,* 13 (5): 219–226.

Neill, M, Hayward, KS and Peterson, T (2007) Students' perceptions of the interprofessional team in practice through the application of servant leadership principles. *Journal of Interprofessional Care,* 21 (4): 425–432. Available from: http://search.ebscohost.com/login.aspx?direct=true&db=rzh&AN=2009652879&site=ehost-live (accessed 2 September 2013).

Newnham, D (2012) Old age giggles. *Nursing Standard,* 27 (5): 25–26.

NHS Choices (2013) *Eat Well Over 60.* Available from: http://www.nhs.uk/Livewell/over60s/Pages/Nutritionover60.aspx (accessed 29 July 2013).

NHS Confederation (2012) *Transforming Patient Experience: The essential guide.* Available from: http://www.institute.nhs.uk/patient_experience/guide/what_matters_to_patients%3f.html (accessed 29 July 2013).

NHS National Patient Safety Agency (2007) *Slips, Trips and Falls in Hospital.* London: NPSA.

Nicholson, N (2012) A review of social isolation: An important but underassessed condition in older adults. *Journal of Primary Prevention,* 33: 137–152.

Nigam, Y and Knight, J (2008a) Exploring the anatomy and physiology of ageing. Part 3 – The digestive system. *Nursing Times,* 104 (33). Available from: www.nursingtimes.net (accessed 2 September 2013).

Nigam, Y and Knight, J (2008b) Exploring the anatomy and physiology of ageing. Part 6 – The eye and ear. *Nursing Times,* 104 (36). Available from: www.nursingtimes.net (accessed 2 September 2013).

Nolan, M, Davies, S and Brown, J (2006a) Transitions in care homes: Towards relationship-centred care using the 'senses framework'. *Quality in Ageing,* 7 (3): 5–14.

Nolan, MR, Brown, J, Davies, S, Nolan, J and Keady, J (2006b) *The Senses Framework: Improving care for older people through a relationship-centred approach.* Getting Research into Practice (GRiP) report no. 2. Project report. Sheffield: University of Sheffield.

Norman, I and Ryrie, I (2009) *The Art and Science of Mental Health Nursing: A text book of principles and practice.* Maidenhead: McGraw Hill, Open University Press.

NSCSHA (2003) *Independent Inquiry into the Death of David Bennett.* Norfolk: NSCSHA.

Nunney, J, Raynor, DK, Knapp, P and Closs, SJ (2011) How do the attitudes and beliefs of older people and health care professionals impact on the use of multiple-compartment compliance aids? A qualitative study using grounded theory. *Drugs Aging,* 28 (5): 403–414.

Nursing and Midwifery Council (2002) *Practitioner–Client Relationships and the Prevention of Abuse.* London: Nursing Midwifery Council.

Nursing and Midwifery Council (2008a) *Standards for Learning and Assessing.* London: NMC.

Nursing and Midwifery Council (2008b) *The Code: Standards of conduct, performance and ethics for nurses and midwives.* London: NMC.

Nursing and Midwifery Council (2009) *Guidance for the Care of Older People.* London: NMC.

Nursing and Midwifery Council (2010) *NMC Standards for Pre-registration Nursing Education.* London: NMC. Available from: http://standards.nmc-uk.org/PublishedDocuments/Standards%20for%20pre-registration%20nursing%20education%2016082010.pdf (accessed 2 September 2013).

Nursing and Midwifery Council (2011) *Standards for Conduct: Performance ethics for nurses and midwives.* Available from: http://www.nmc-uk.org/Nurses-and-midwives/The-code/The-code-in-full (accessed 2 September 2013).

Nyman, SR, Hogarth, HA, Ballinger, C and Victor, CR (2011) Representations of old age in falls prevention websites: Implications for likely uptake of advice by older people. *British Journal of Occupational Therapy*, 74 (8): 366–374.

O'Keeffe, M, Hills, A, Doyle, M, McCreadie, C, Scholes, S, Constantine, R, Tinker, A, Manthorpe, J, Biggs, S and Erens, B (2007) *UK Study of Abuse and Neglect of Older People Prevalence Survey Report.* London: Comic Relief/Department of Health.

O'Sullivan, G and Hocking, C (2006) Positive ageing in residential care. *New Zealand Journal of Occupational Therapy*, 53 (1): 17–23.

Office for National Statistics (2012a) *Statistical Bulletin 2011 Census: Population estimates for the United Kingdom, 27 March 2011.* Available at: http://www.ons.gov.uk/ons/dcp171778_292378.pdf (accessed 14 August 2013).

Office for National Statistics (2012b) *Video Summary: Ethnicity in England and Wales. Part of 2011 census, key statistics for local authorities in England and Wales release.* Available at: http://www.ons.gov.uk/ons/rel/census/2011-census/key-statistics-for-local-authorities-in-england-and-wales/video-summary-ethnicity.html (accessed 14 August 2013).

Office for National Statistics (2013) *Statistical Bulletin 2011 Census: Quick statistics for England and Wales, March 2011.* Available at: http://www.ons.gov.uk/ons/dcp171778_297002.pdf (accessed 2 September 2013).

Oliver, D (in press) Discrimination in health services for older people (UK). *International Journal of Medical Ethics.*

Oliver, D and Healey, F (2009) Falls risk prediction tools for hospital inpatients: Do they work? *Nursing Times*, 105 (7): 18–21.

Ong, AD, Rothstein, JD and Uchino, BN (2012) Loneliness accentuates age differnces in cardiovascular responses to social evaluation. *Psychology and Aging*, 27 (1): 190–198.

Orchard, CA and Bainbridge, LA (2010) *A National Interprofessional Competency Framework.* Vancouver: Canadian Interprofessional Health Collaborative.

Parliamentary and Health Service Ombudsman (2011) *Care and Compassion?* London: Parliamentary and Health Service Ombudsman.

Parliamentary Office for Science and Technology (2007) *Postnote: Ethnicity and health.* Available at: http://www.parliament.uk/documents/post/postpn276.pdf (accessed 2 September 2013).

Patient Safety First (2009) *The 'How To' Guide for Reducing Harm from Falls.* Available from: http://www.patientsafetyfirst.nhs.uk (accessed 2 September 2013).

Patients Association (2009) *Patients ... Not Numbers, People ... Not Statistics.* London: Patients Association. Available from: http://www.patients-association.com/Portals/0/Public/Files/Research%20Publications/Patients%20not%20numbers,%20people%20not%20statistics.pdf (accessed 2 September 2013).

Patients Association (2011a) *We've Been Listening, Have You Been Learning?* London: Patients Association. Available from: http://www.patients-association.com/Portals/0/We've%20been%20listening,%20have%20you%20been%20learning.pdf (accessed 29 July 2013).

Patients Association (2011b) *Listen to Patients, Speak up for Change.* London: Patients Association. Available from: http://www.patients-association.com/Portals/0/Public/Files/Research%20 Publications/Listen%20to%20patients,%20Speak%20up%20for%20change.pdf (accessed 29 July 2013).

Pearcey, P (2010) Caring? It's the little things we are not supposed to do anymore. *International Journal of Nursing Practice,* 16 (1): 51–56.

Peate, I (2003) Medicines and the older person: Principles of good practice. *British Journal of Nursing,* 12 (9): 530–535.

Pellatt, GC (2006) The role of mentors in supporting pre-registration nursing students. *British Journal of Nursing,* 15 (6): 336–340.

Penhale, B and Parker, J (2008) *Working with Vulnerable Adults.* London: Routledge.

Peplau, LA and Perlman, D (eds) (1982) *Loneliness: A sourcebook of current theory, research, and therapy.* New York: Wiley-Interscience.

Phillips, L (2013) Delirium in geriatric patients: Identification and prevention. *MEDSURG Nursing,* 22 (1): 9–13.

Phinney, A (2008) Understanding experiences of dementia. In: Downes, M and Bowers, B (eds) *Excellence in Dementia Care.* London: McGraw Hill.

Plan UK (2013) *Help End Forced Marriage.* Available at: http://www.plan-uk.org/what-we-do/ campaigns/because-i-am-a-girl/get-involved/girls-fund/plan-for-girls (accessed 2 September 2013).

Pressman, S and Cohen, S (2005) Does positive affect influence health? *Psychological Bulletin,* 131: 925–971.

Price, E (2005) All but invisible: Older gay men and lesbians. *Nursing Older People,* 17 (4): 16–18.

Prudential (2011) *Class of 2011 Study.* London: Prudential. Available from: http://www.prweb. com/pdfdownload/4997394.pdf (accessed 30 August 2011).

Putnam, R (2000) *Bowling Alone: The collapse and revival of American community.* New York: Simon and Schuster.

Rayner, G (2009) Conventional and ecological public health. *Public Health,* 123: 587e91.

Raynes, N, Clark, H and Beecham, J (eds) (2006) *The Report of the Older People's Inquiry into 'That Bit of Help'.* Joseph Rowntree Foundation. Available from: http://www.jrf.org.uk/sites/files/jrf/ briefing03.pdf (accessed 2 September 2013).

Reed, J, Cook, G, Childs, S and Hall, A (2003) *'Getting Old Is Not for Cowards': Comfortable, healthy, aging.* York: Joseph Rowntree Foundation.

Rees, K (2007) Growing old is no gradual decline. *Working With Older People,* 11 (4): 28–31.

Reid, J (2012) Clinical human factors: The need to speak up to improve patient safety. *Online,* 26 (35): 35–40.

Richardson, GE (2002) Mental health promotion through resilience and resiliency education. *Journal of Emergency Mental Health,* 4: 65–75.

Ritzer, G (ed.) (2007) *Blackwell Encyclopedia of Sociology.* Oxford: Blackwell Publishing.

Rogers, A (1997) Vulnerability, health and healthcare. *Journal of Advanced Nursing,* 26: 65–72.

Rogers, CR (1951) *Client Centred Therapy.* London: Constable.

Rogers, S (2010) *England and Wales' Population Broken Down by Race, Sex, Age and Place.* Available at: http://www.theguardian.com/news/datablog/2010/feb/26/population-ethnic-race-age-statistics (accessed 14 August 2013).

Rondahl, G, Innala, S and Carlsson, M (2006) Heterosexual assumptions in verbal and non-verbal communication in nursing. *Journal of Advanced Nursing,* 56 (4): 373–381.

Routsalo, PE, Tilvis, RS, Kautiainen, H and Pitkala, KH (2009) Effects of psychosocial group rehabilitation on social functioning, loneliness, and wellbeing of lonely older people: Randomized controlled trial. *Journal of Advanced Nursing,* 65: 297–305.

Royal College of Nursing (2008) *An Ageing Population: Education and practice preparation for nursing students learning to work with older people.* London: RCN.

Royal College of Physicians (2007) *The Assessment of Pain in Older People.* Available from: http://www.britishpainsociety.org/book_pain_older_people.pdf (accessed 2 September 2013).

Royal College of Psychiatrists (2005) *Who Cares Wins: Guidelines for the development of liaison mental health services for older people.* London: RCP.

Rungapadiachy, D (1999) *Interpersonal Communications and Psychology for Health Care Professionals.* Oxford: Butterworth Heinemann.

Rydeman, I and Törnkvist, L (2006) The patients' vulnerability, dependence and exposed situation in the discharge process: Experiences of district nurses, geriatric nurses and social workers. *Journal of Clinical Nursing,* 15: 1299–1307.

Sabat, S, Johnson, A, Swarbrick, C and Keady, J (2011) The 'demented other' or simply 'a person'? Extending the philosophical discourse of Naue and Kroll though the situated self. *Nursing Philosophy,* 12: 282–292.

Saczynski, JS, Pfeifer, L, Masaki, K, Korf, ESC, Laurin, D, White, L et al. (2006) The effect of social engagement on incident dementia: The Honolulu-Asia Aging Study. *American Journal of Epidemiology,* 163: 433–440.

Salari, S (2005) Intergenerational partnerships in adult day centres: Importance of age-appropriate environments and behaviors. *The Gerontologist,* 42 (3): 321–333.

Scammell, J and Olumide, G (2012) Racism and the mentor–student relationship: Nurse education through a white lens. *Nurse Education Today,* 32: 545–550.

Scammell, J, Hemingway, A and Heaslip, V (2012) Humanising values at the heart of nurse education. *Nursing Times,* 108 (41): 26–28.

Scotland.gov (2010) *Alcohol and its Impact on Health.* Available from: http://www.scotland.gov.uk/Topics/Health/health/Alcohol/health (accessed 2 September 2013).

Scott, J and Marshall, G (2009) *A Dictionary of Sociology.* Oxford: OUP.

Shapiro, D, West, MA, Borrill, CS, Carletta, J, Carter, AJ, Dawson, JF, Garrod, S et al. (2001) *The Effectiveness of Health Care Teams in the National Health Service.* Birmingham: Department of Health.

Shepherd, G, Boardman, J and Slade, M (2008) *Making Recovery a Reality: A policy document.* London: Sainsbury Centre for Mental Health.

Social Care Institute for Excellence (2005) *Update for SCIE Best Practice Guide Assessing the Mental Health Needs of Older People.* Available from: http://www.scie.org.uk/publications/guides/guide03/files/research.pdf (accessed 2 September 2013).

Social Care Institute for Excellence (2007) *Assessing the Mental Health Needs of Older People: Mental health and wellbeing.* SCIE guide 3. Available from: http://www.scie.org.uk/publications/guides/guide03/framework/wellbeing.asp (accessed 2 September 2013).

Social Care Institute for Excellence (2012) *Preventing Loneliness and Social Isolation in Older People.* Available from: http://www.scie.org.uk/publications/ataglance/ataglance60.pdf (accessed 2 September 2013).

Sørlie, V, Torjuul, K, Ross, A and Kihlgren, M (2006) Satisfied patients are also vulnerable patients: Narratives from an acute care ward. *Journal of Clinical Nursing,* 15 (15): 1240–1246.

Soule, A, Babb, P, Evandrou, M, Balchin S and Zealey, LL (2005) *Focus on Older People.* Newport: Office of National Statistics.

Spiers, J (2000) New perspectives on vulnerability using emic and etic approaches. *Journal of Advanced Nursing,* 31 (3): 715–721.

Stanley, M, Moyle, W, Ballantyne, A, Jaworski, K, Corlis, M, Oxlade, D, Stoll, A and Young, B (2010) Nowadays you don't even see your neighbours: Loneliness in the everyday lives of older Australians. *Health and Social Care in the Community,* 18 (4): 407–414.

Stansfeld, SA, Fuhrer, R, Shipley, MJ and Marmot, M (2002) Psychological distress as a risk factor for CHD in the Whitehall II study. *International Journal of Epidemiology,* 31: 248e55.

Stenbock-Hult, B and Sarvimäki, A (2011) The meaning of vulnerability to nurses caring for older people. *Nursing Ethics,* 18 (1): 31–41.

Stephan, B and Brayne, C (2008) Prevalence and projections of dementia. In Downs, M and Bowers, B (eds.) *Excellence in Dementia Care, Research into Practice.* Maidenhead: McGraw Hill, Open University Press.

Stickley, T (2011) From SOLER to SURETY for effective non-verbal communication. *Nurse Education in Practice,* 11 (6): 395–398.

Stockwell, F (1972) *The Unpopular Patient.* London: Royal College of Nursing.

Tanner, D and Harris, J (2008) *Working with Older People.* London: Routledge.

Taylor, C, Lillis, C, LeMone, P and Lynn, P (2011) *Fundamentals of Nursing: The art and science of nursing care,* 7th edn. London: Lippincott Williams and Wilkins.

The Economist (2010) The U bend of life. 16 December 2010. Available from: http://www.economist.com/node/17722567 (accessed 2 September 2013).

Thompson, N (1998) *Promoting Equality: Challenging discrimination and oppression in the human services.* London: Macmillan.

Thornley, C (2000) A question of competence? Re-evaluating the roles of the nursing auxiliary and health care assistant in the NHS. *Journal of Clinical Nursing,* 9 (3): 451–458. Available from: http://www.ncbi.nlm.nih.gov/pubmed/11235321 (accessed 2 September 2013).

Thornton, JE (2002) Myths of aging or ageist stereotypes. *Educational Gerontology*, 28: 301–312.

Tillich, P (2002) *The Eternal Now*. London: SCM.

Todres, L, Galvin, K and Holloway, I (2009) The humanisation of health care: A value framework for qualitative research. *International Journal of Qualitative Studies on Health and Wellbeing*, 4: 66–77.

Tomaka, J, Thompson, S and Palacios, R (2006) The relation of social isolation, loneliness, and social support to disease outcomes among the elderly. *Journal of Aging and Health*, 18: 359–384.

Trivedi, D, Goodman, C, Gage, H, Baron, N, Scheibi, F, Lliffe, S, Manthorpe, J et al. (2012) The effectiveness of inter-professional working for older people living in the community: A systematic review. *Health and Social Care in the Community*, 1–16. Available from: http://www.ncbi.nlm.nih.gov/pubmed/22891915 (accessed 6 December 2012).

Tuckman, BW (1965) Developmental sequence in small groups. *Psychological Bulletin*, 63: 384–399.

Uhlenberg, P and Miner, S (1996) Life course and aging. In: Binstock, RH and George, LK (eds) *Handbook of Aging and the Social Sciences*. San Diego, CA: Academic Press, pp. 208–228.

United Nations (2012) *Population Ageing and Development 2012*. Available from: http://www.un.org/esa/population/publications/2012WorldPopAgeingDev_Chart/2012PopAgeingandDev_WallChart.pdf (accessed 8 April 2013).

van Baarsen, B, Snijders, TAB, Smit, JH and van Duijn, MAJ (2001) Lonely but not alone: Emotional isolation and social isolation as two distinct dimensions of loneliness in older people. *Educational and Psychological Measurement*, 61: 119–135.

Van der Elst, E, Dierclox de Casterle, B and Gastmans, C (2012) Elderly patients' and residents' perceptions of 'the good nurse': A literature review. *Journal of Medical Ethics*, 38 (2): 93–97.

Victor, C (2005) *The Social Context of Ageing: A textbook of gerontology*. London: Routledge.

Vincenzi, H and Grabosky, F (1987) Measuring the emotional and social aspects of loneliness and isolation. *Journal of Social Behavior and Personality*, 2: 257–270.

Wade, DT and Halligan, PW (2004) Do biomedical models of illness made for good health care system? *British Medical Journal*, 329 (7479): 1398.

Wagg, A, Potter, J, Peel, P, Irwin, P, Lowe, D and Pearson, M (2008) National audit of continence care for older people: Management of urinary incontinence. *Age and Ageing*, 37: 39–44.

Wagnild, GM and Young, HM (1990) Resilience among older women. *Image Journal Nursing*, 22 (4): 252–255.

Wakefield, A, Spilsbury, K, Atkin, K and McKenna, H (2010) What work do assistant practitioners do and where do they fit in the nursing workforce? *Nursing Times*, 106: 12.

Ward, R, Howorth, M, Wilkinson, H, Campbell, S and Keady, J (2011) Supporting the friendships of people with dementia. Available online at: http://dem.sagepub.com/content/early/2011/10/05/1471301211421064 (accessed October 2011).

Williams, K, Kemper, S and Hummert, ML (2004) Enhancing communication with older adults: Overcoming elderspeak. *Journal of Gerontological Nursing*, Oct: 17–25.

Williamson, T (2011) Grouchy old men? Promoting older men's mental health and emotional wellbeing. *Working with Older People*, 15 (4): 164–176.

Wilson, RS, Krueger, KR, Arnold, SE et al. (2007) Loneliness and risk of Alzheimer's disease. *Archives of General Psychiatry*, 64: 234–240.

Wood, V and Robertson, JF (1978) Friendship and kinship interaction: Differential effect on morale of the elderly. *Journal of Marriage and the Family*, 40 (2): 367–375.

Woolhead, G, Calnan, M, Dieppe, P and Tadd, W (2004) Dignity in older age: What do older people in the UK think? *Age and Ageing*, 33: 165–270.

Worden, A, Challis, DJ and Pedersen, I (2005) The assessment of older people's needs in care homes. *Aging and Mental Health*, 10 (5): 549–557.

World Health Organization (2002) *Active Aging: A policy framework*. Available from: http://www.who.int/hpr/ageing/ActiveAgeingPolicyFrame.pdf (accessed 2 September 2013).

World Health Organization (2004) *Active Ageing: Towards age-friendly primary health care*. Geneva: WHO.

World Health Organization (2007a) *Global Age-Friendly Cities: A guide*. France: World Health Organization. Available from: http://www.who.int/ageing/publications/Global_age_friendly_cities_Guide_English.pdf (accessed 2 September 2013).

World Health Organization (2007b) *What is Mental Health*? Available from: http://www.who.int/features/qa/62/en/index.html (accessed 2 September 2013).

World Health Organization (2007c) *WHO Global Report on Falls Prevention in Older Age*. Geneva: WHO.

World Health Organization (2008) *International Health Regulations*, 2nd edn. Geneva: World Health Organization.

World Health Organization (2010a) *Framework for Action on Interprofessional Education and Collaborative Practice*. Geneva: WHO.

World Health Organization (2010b) *International Classification of Diseases – 10*. Available from: http://apps.who.int/classifications/icd10/browse/2010/en#/F00-F09 (accessed 2 September 2013).

World Health Organization (2011) *Global Health and Aging*. Available from: http://www.who.int/ageing/publications/global_health/en/index.html (accessed 29 July 2013).

World Health Organization (2013a) *Infection Prevention and Control in Health Care*. Available from: http://www.who.int/csr/bioriskreduction/infection_control/en/index.html (accessed 29 July 2013).

World Health Organization (2013b) Definition of an older or elderly person. Available from: http://www.who.int/healthinfo/survey/ageingdefnolder/en (accessed 8 April 2013).

Wray, S (2003) Women growing older: Agency, ethnicity and culture. *Sociology*, 37 (3): 511–527.

Yuval-Davis, N (2006) Intersectionality and feminist politics. *European Journal of Women's Studies*, 13 (3): 193–209.

Index